Advance Praise for *10 Lessons in Public Health*

"Part treatise on how to be an outstanding public health leader and part adventure novel. Sommer shares the defining moments that changed his own career and the global health landscape."

—Pierre Buekens, M.D.,
W. H. Watkins Professor and Dean,
Department of Epidemiology,
Tulane University School of Public Health
and Tropical Medicine

"Al Sommer has distilled a lifetime of experience, adventure, and leadership into ten key lessons for aspiring leaders in public health. What Albert Schweitzer once observed about himself this book reveals about Alfred Sommer: his life is his argument. Sommer's life story lays out the case in a lively, readable, compelling, and inspirational way."

—Harvey V. Fineberg, M.D., Ph.D., President,
Institute of Medicine

"This personal global health journey by a blazing pioneer in the field—through cholera, smallpox, blindness, a cyclone, and civil war—is an inspiring read for those considering a career in global health. It illustrates what can be done through perseverance and a passion to make a difference."

—Michael H. Merson, M.D., Founding Director,
Duke Global Health Institute

"Dr. Sommer observes that pursuing global health requires one 'to stray from the traditional path.' For those of us making this leap, he offers both inspiration and challenge. Inspiration that the less trodden path will yield the greatest

societal impact and personal joy. And a challenge to pursue such a path ethically, tenaciously, inquisitively, and irreverently."
—Rebecca Onie, J.D., Cofounder and CEO, Health Leads

"Dr. Sommer's book makes the central point that a single person can fundamentally transform the lives of millions through a collision of intellect, serendipity, zeal for discovery, and respect for data. This is an engaging story to be read by every student of science and medicine—at the very least.

"Dr. Sommer's trek begins in cholera-ridden, postcolonial East Pakistan and concludes at Johns Hopkins. Along the way, his scientific insights and zeal lead to some of the most impactful discoveries of our time—including saving the sight and lives of millions of children.

"His career has been spent, although sometimes serendipitously and not without self-deprecating humor, doing things 'that matter.' His is 'meaningful science' with a direct and immediate human impact and a story that should be read."
—David W. Parke II, M.D.,
Executive Vice President and CEO,
American Academy of Ophthalmology

"Through an often humorous account of his unique early personal trajectory, Al Sommer provides down-to-earth and inspiring advice for anybody interested in global health, for whom this book is the ultimate career guide."
—Peter Piot, C.M.G., M.D., Ph.D., D.T.M., F.R.C.P.,
F.Med.Sci., former UNAIDS Executive Director,
former Under Secretary-General of the United Nations,
Director of the London School
of Hygiene and Tropical Medicine

"The Centers for Disease Control and Prevention would find this book extremely useful in the training of its EIS officers. There are few, if any, similar publications written by a person with the experience and accomplishments of Dr. Sommer."
> —Harrison C. Spencer, M.D., M.P.H.,
> President and CEO,
> Association of Schools of Public Health

"Al Sommer is as good a story teller as he is an epidemiologist and ophthalmologist. His stories are riveting, insightful, and inspiring. This most enjoyable read summarizes the life of a man who has taken many forks in the road, with nearly universal productivity in all."
> —Bruce E. Spivey, M.D., M.Ed., M.S.,
> Chairman, Pacific Vision Foundation,
> President of the International Council of Ophthalmology

"There is a limit to what can be learned in a classroom about how to succeed in global public health. Al Sommer, fittingly, takes us into the field, tracing ten great lessons in public health practice learned through the trials, triumphs, mistakes, and wonderful surprises he encountered on his own path from Bangladesh to Baltimore."
> —Emily Vasquez, Ph.D. candidate,
> Department of Sociomedical Sciences,
> Columbia University

10 LESSONS IN PUBLIC HEALTH

10 LESSONS
IN PUBLIC HEALTH
Inspiration for Tomorrow's Leaders

ALFRED SOMMER, M.D., M.H.S.

The Johns Hopkins University Press

Baltimore

© 2013 The Johns Hopkins University Press
All rights reserved. Published 2013
Printed in the United States of America on acid-free paper
9 8 7 6 5 4 3 2

The Johns Hopkins University Press
2715 North Charles Street
Baltimore, Maryland 21218-4363
www.press.jhu.edu

Library of Congress Cataloging-in-Publication Data

Sommer, Alfred, 1942–
   Ten lessons in public health : inspiration for tomorrow's leaders /
Alfred Sommer.
       p. ; cm.
   ISBN 978-1-4214-0952-8 (hardcover : alk. paper) — ISBN 1-4214-0952-6
(hardcover : alk. paper) — ISBN 978-1-4214-0904-7 (pbk. : alk. paper) — ISBN
1-4214-0904-6 (pbk. : alk. paper) — ISBN 978-1-4214-0905-4 (electronic) —
ISBN 1-4214-0905-4 (electronic)
       I. Title.
   [DNLM: 1. Sommer, Alfred, 1942– 2. Epidemiology—United States—
Autobiography. 3. International Cooperation—United States—Autobiography.
4. World Health—United States—Autobiography. WZ 100]

       362.1092'273—dc23   2012035330

A catalog record for this book is available from the British Library.

All photographs are the author's.

*Special discounts are available for bulk purchases of this book. For more
information, please contact Special Sales at 410-516-6936 or specialsales@
press.jhu.edu.*

The Johns Hopkins University Press uses environmentally friendly book
materials, including recycled text paper that is composed of at least 30 percent
post-consumer waste, whenever possible.

To Jill, Charles, and Marni
(Who put up with it all)

and

To the families of those who are
entering careers in global public health
(For all they might eventually put up with)

Contents

IIIIIIIIIIIIIIIIIIIIIIIIIIIIIIIIIIIIIIIIIIIIIIIIIIIIIIIIIIIIIIIIIIIIIIIIIIIIIIIIIIIIIIIIIIIIIIIIIIIIIIIIIIIIIIIIIIIIIIIIIIIIIIIIIIIIIIIIIIIIIIIIIIIIIIIIIIIIIIIII

Preface

Research is formalized curiosity.

ZORA NEALE HURSTON

"Global health" now attracts the interest of the press, the World Economic Forum, and young people everywhere—undergraduate and graduate students, physicians, nurses, health managers, and public health professionals of every stripe. It has become the destination major of many applicants to university schools of arts and sciences, medicine, nursing, and public health, especially the Bloomberg School of Public Health at Johns Hopkins. Undergraduates on campuses across America (and in many other countries around the world) are editing and publishing slick magazines devoted to the subject, while every major academic institution worth its salt has established programs, departments, or institutes of "global health." Yet the term itself is barely a decade old.

How did this suddenly happen? It wasn't sudden. Many people have been laboring in these fields for half a century or more. We've been tackling diseases, new and old, by identifying their causes and determinants, devising and testing programs for their control, and attempting to convince policymakers of the importance of vigorous, evidence-based interventions.

What has changed, for a multiplicity of reasons, is the attention these pursuits now receive, the importance they are accorded, and the passion with which a new generation has embraced their cause. What's now called "global health" is traditional "public health" writ large: public health explicitly played out, as it always has been, on the global stage. But the new terminology graphically reminds us that no population can feel smugly safe while others are ill, whether from infectious diseases like SARS, influenza, tuberculosis, or HIV/AIDS, or from chronic (often behaviorally "communicable") diseases like obesity, stroke, and chronic obstructive pulmonary disease. While genes are important, they don't explain, nor are they responsible for, the epidemics of lung cancer, diabetes, and asthma that are now sweeping the globe.

Many disciplines contribute to the design and conduct of successful global health interventions, but success almost always begins with the classic epidemiologic triangulation of a disease by time, place, and person. Why this person and not the person next door; why now and not last week or next year? Epidemiologic investigations and insights provide the evidence behind good medical practice and global (public) health policy.

We epidemiologists have been handed powerful new tools to assist our work, from laboratory tests that identify new infectious agents to powerful computers that can quickly carry out complex analyses. But nothing can replace epidemiology's core underpinnings: the rigorous collection of data and their thoughtful, innovative interrogation. "Connecting the dots" is what matters most.

I've had the good fortune of being able to follow my interests (and enhance my ability to connect the dots) by chasing down a diverse array of global health threats. Sometimes these efforts led to insights that were not particularly relevant—until they were, urgently, forty years later. At other times they led to discoveries that launched global programs that now save the sight and lives of millions of people. In one instance, my own work, in a small way, helped to establish a new nation.

Any significant involvement in global health demands a willingness to stray from the traditional path—on your part and that of your spouse or partner. I've known few instances in which a global (public) health career wasn't supported by a joint interest in experiencing other environments and engaging with other cultures.

This small treatise tells of my immersion in a world where data mattered mightily but persistence, powers of persuasion, and luck mattered nearly as much. It is my hope that these personal stories will help those considering careers in global health to better appreciate—through my successes and failures, frustrations and celebrations, plans and accidents—how interesting and unpredictable epidemiology and a life immersed in global health can be, and how much our individual contributions can matter.

I hope that this brief retelling of moments along my personal journey will help you in yours.

My own journey was influenced by many marvelously supportive mentors and role models, among them, Howard Hiatt, George Comstock, Abe Lilienfeld, Helen Abbey, Ed Maumenee, Arnall Patz, Alex Languire, and Bill Foege—all luminaries in the annals of medicine and global public health. I am grateful to them all. Those eager to make a difference in the world will do well to read about these mentors. (But more important, find your own.) My immediate thanks go to the Rockefeller Foundation's Bellagio Center, which generously provided tranquil space in which to recollect these thoughts.

I am deeply indebted to Vincent J. Burke for encouraging my preparation of this book, and for editing out two-thirds of my initial manuscript and improving on the remainder.

10 LESSONS IN PUBLIC HEALTH

GO WHERE THE PROBLEMS ARE

The world is very different now. For man holds in his
mortal hands the power to abolish all forms of human poverty and all forms of human life.

JOHN F. KENNEDY

llllllllllllllllllllllllllllllllllllllllllllllllllllllllllllllllllllllllllllllllllllllllllllllllllllllllllllllllllllllllllllllllllllllllllllllllllllllllllll

Inspired during medical school by John F. Kennedy's
framing of the choices for my generation, my wife,
Jill, and I decided that once my training was completed we
would serve in the Peace Corps.

Three years later, much had changed. With a year of
medical residency still to go, I received an official letter from
the Peace Corps informing me that Congress had passed
new legislation. I was told I would be drafted out of the
Peace Corps and sent to Vietnam. The change between the
Kennedy inauguration and the Johnson era was dramatic.

Going to Vietnam was the last thing I wanted to do. I
hastily nabbed one of the few "draft-fulfilling positions" still
available to physicians, by enrolling in the EIS (Epidemic Intelligence Service) at the Centers for Disease Control (CDC)
in Atlanta. My future life, interests, and career were set on a
course I had little anticipated.

Those directing the CDC unit to which I was initially
assigned were considerably less energetically engaged than

I'd grown accustomed to. They, in turn, concluded that my "constant need for new challenges" (as they put it) was a pain in their collective necks. I was sent home for two weeks to "relax," which suited me fine, since our first child was about to be born. When I returned, I discovered that another EIS unit, stationed at the Cholera Research Laboratory (CRL) in what was then called East Pakistan, was fully engaged and excited by their work, and they happened at that moment to be looking for an epidemiologist. I quickly volunteered and, along with Jill and our new son, Charles, soon joined this U.S. effort to contain the spread of cholera.

To me, this seemed an ideal opportunity: an intellectually engaging overseas cultural experience without becoming part of the Vietnam tragedy. We were young, idealistic, eager, and more than a little naïve. Little did we know that we would be caught up in a cyclone disaster that would wash away a quarter of a million people in one night, a civil war that would produce ten million refugees and give birth to a new nation, and a smallpox epidemic that would go down in the annals of medical history.

In April 1970, we arrived in Dacca (now Dhaka), East Pakistan (now Bangladesh), in the Bengal region of the Indian subcontinent, with Charles (5 months old) in tow. Except for a honeymoon camping through Europe, our lives until then had been pretty narrowly circumscribed.

Dacca was not a particularly attractive place. It was extremely hot and humid, possessed only one restaurant patronized by foreigners, and had only a few, second-rate tourist attractions. People, cows, chickens, bicycles, buses, and the occasional car jostled each other on the streets, particularly in the warrens of Old Dacca. The poverty was extreme and pervasive. The best that could be (and often was) said about Dacca was that it was "equally close to all the places you'd rather be" (if where you'd rather be happened to be in South Asia).

Despite its pervasive poverty and sporadic electricity service, Dacca was not a difficult place for expatriates. Like most of my colleagues at the Cholera Research Laboratory, we lived in a quiet suburb at the periphery of town, where coconut trees soared above each family's walled compound. Outside the walls, emaciated cows and mangy dogs wandered the dusty streets. For the middle-class Bengalis living in the neighborhood, the streets and lanes outside the walls were like unrelated entities on another planet—the place where your banana peel landed when you tossed it over your compound's wall.

We occupied a large house with a sweeping verandah that came with seven air conditioners and six servants. For two middle-class American liberals, six servants took some getting used to. In truth, we were not so lavishly waited upon as their numbers might suggest: the highly stratified caste system dictated that the cook not clean the dishes, and that the driver not wash the car. The sweeper disposed of the garbage, the chowkidar maintained the garden, the bearer laundered the linen, and the ayah bathed Charles.

The house we inherited from my predecessor was first rate; the servants that accompanied it were not, but what did we know? It was tough enough just *having* "servants." After a month or so, friends began asking why we were putting up with such terrible staff—hadn't we known that the best servants are always hired away when someone departs, leaving the rejects to be passed along with the house? "But how can we fire someone who needs a job?" we asked. "You can," we were told, "because there are twenty-two million unemployed Bengalis who would love these jobs and deserve them more." It took another month, and innumerable awkward moments, before Jill and I could muster sufficient courage to act on this perfectly sensible principle. We eventually acquired a group of hard-working, pleasant staff who earned their keep.

At that time, most career Foreign Service officers considered an assignment to Dacca penance for time they'd spent at embassies in London or Rome, but for those of us only a few years out of medical school it was an exotic adventure. Giant ceiling fans in every room, expansive gardens filled with exotic fruit trees, dinner parties that revolved around the latest political intrigue. We were living the ultimate Humphrey Bogart flick, minus, for the moment, melodramatic conflicts.

Dacca gave real meaning to that oft-cited—but only vaguely appreciated—phrase, "a moonless night." Jon Rohde, a medical school classmate and his wife, Candy, occupied the compound immediately adjacent to ours. A large welcome party had been organized for the night we arrived. After showering, we took Charles in our arms and walked through the gate of our compound. Within ten feet we were hopelessly lost. It was so dark we could not see their house next door, and we could only barely see the ground we were walking on. We never again ventured out on moonless nights without a flashlight.

We had never given a thought to the fact that we were Jewish and Pakistan was overwhelmingly Muslim. To our amusement, we discovered that the average villager assumed that any foreigner was Christian. Our Pakistani colleagues knew better, and to them our religious persuasion turned out to be a great advantage. Jill insisted that we keep Kosher at home, to the degree possible, which in Pakistan meant no pork in the house. News of this idiosyncrasy quickly got around. Muslim colleagues, who would attend receptions but rarely dinners at foreigners' homes, regularly accepted our invitations to dine. Our invitations had initially been extended out of courtesy, not with any expectation that people would attend (because we'd been warned by our expatriate friends that they wouldn't). But, being Kosher, our food was also Halal, adhering to the same pork-free attributes stipulated by Islam.

We had settled in, far from home and family, on the other side of the world. We had gone to a place where "the problems" were. Many big problems, as it turned out.

GET INTO THE FIELD

A problem must be such that it matters what the answer is—whether to science generally or to mankind.

PETER MEDAWAR

W hile our home was in Dacca, my work was "in the
field." I wasn't sent to Pakistan to live the good
life in a compound but to learn how cholera, that rapidly
lethal diarrheal disease, spread and to test new vaccines to
prevent it. Cholera would occasionally break out of its histor-
ical home, the fetid delta regions of the Indian subcontinent.
Such was the case in the 1960s. Sporadic outbreaks began
occurring elsewhere in Asia, and also in Africa and even the
Americas. U.S. health planners were concerned that it might
be only a matter of time before cholera invaded the United
States.

With our Southeast Asia Treaty Organization (SEATO)
allies, the United States had created a major research program at the Cholera Research Laboratory (CRL) in East
Pakistan. Its headquarters, laboratory, and main hospital
were located in Dacca, the capital; a field hospital and study
population of 250,000 were centered on Matlab Bazaar, a
rural market town. The trip there took one hour in a hot,

cramped, un-air-conditioned Chevrolet Blazer, plus three hours—far more pleasant—by speedboat. On those car rides I silently cursed the stateside bureaucrat who, never having worked in the tropics, saved a couple hundred dollars by buying the program a vehicle without air conditioning and with only two doors (and thus only two windows to roll down).

CRL was staffed by Bengali and (largely U.S.) expatriate scientists. Half were employed by the National Institutes of Health (NIH), to study the mechanisms by which cholera infection caused dehydrating diarrhea, and half by the CDC, to test the effectiveness of cholera vaccines.

The villages around Matlab Bazaar were, quite literally, dirt poor. Except for a rare wooden house or tin roof, almost all the homes were made of mud and daub, with thatched roofs. The poorer homes were always crumbling (the mud walls needed to be replaced annually after the monsoon rains). None of the dwellings had running water. Cows, chickens, water buffalo, and goats competed with humans for living space. The only sources of truly potable water were occasional (and only occasionally working) hand-pumped artesian wells. Most drinking water was drawn from polluted ponds and open wells.

Despite their profound poverty, the villages were startlingly neat and clean. Each species of animal (excepting the chickens) occupied its own place. Human waste was deposited in the fields or at the edge of a pond, never in the living areas. The floors of the huts were under constant maintenance, kept smooth by regular applications of fresh mud.

The entire study population was carefully monitored for diarrhea; any suspected cases of cholera were quickly transported by speedboat to the Matlab hospital. In cases of cholera, time is of the essence. The diarrhea that is cholera's hallmark can rapidly dehydrate a patient, resulting in coma and cardiovascular collapse within hours. Patients routinely arrived at the hospital having lost more than 10 percent of their body weight. Shriveled and shrunken, with a barely perceptible pulse, they often appeared dead on arrival, but replacing lost body fluids quickly revived them, convincing more than one villager that we literally raised people from the dead. Possibly my saddest experiences were the times I had to explain to distraught mothers, who often had traveled great distances carrying unresponsive children in their arms, that we did not perform miracles and could not bring their dead son or daughter back to life.

At that time the available cholera vaccines were entirely useless, yet national authorities throughout the developing world insisted that all visitors be vaccinated before they entered the country. There being no viable vaccine worth testing—one of the program's assignments—I instead investigated the ways in which cholera spread, hoping to find clues that might tell us how to stop it early. This was classical epidemiology.

One of the first things I wondered about was whether the regular use of pathogen-free artesian well water (when available), instead of inevitably polluted local pond water, really lessened the risk of contracting cholera (as one might expect, but should never assume without testing). Billy Woodward, the CDC epidemiologist who had preceded me, spent three years carefully recording every case of cholera in the Matlab field area. This produced hard-to-come-by longitudinal study data. It also proved to be an important lesson—if you can save the effort of collecting your own data by using someone else's, by all means do so, as long as you are convinced the data were rigorously collected and are reliable.

Given that I did not believe I could obtain a reliable history of each family's artesian-well use, particularly over a three-year period, I reasoned that the distance between a home and the nearest functioning "tube well" might serve as a valid surrogate for such use. Since we already had the longitudinal data on three years of cholera frequency, I had field workers map each house and tube well and plot the distance between them. This was a grossly simplified investigation fraught with unwarranted assumptions, but it was also the first epidemiologic study I had ever undertaken and the first time, as far as I could determine, that anyone had posed this seemingly basic question. (And I was quite taken with my clever use of data painfully collected over many years by someone else!) It turned out that proximity to a functioning tube well reduced the risk of contracting the Classical/Inaba strain of cholera by 85 percent, but it had no impact whatsoever on transmission of the newer, El Tor Ogawa strain. Increasing the number and distribution of working tube wells, it seemed, might help to reduce the commonest strain of cholera. (UNICEF [United Nations International Children's Emergency Fund] subsequently embarked on a major, seemingly successful tube well construction program—only to discover, after the fact, that in many areas the water contained unacceptable levels of naturally occurring arsenic.)

Of course, most often you need to get out into the field and collect your own data (occasionally—if not predictably—at considerable personal risk). We learned of a cholera epidemic, caused by a new strain of bacteria, which had broken out in Rangpur district, far north of our treatment facilities. To study its epidemiologic and clinical profile, and to provide local relief, we established a makeshift clinic in an old house in the affected area and took turns staffing the facility and treating its patients. Mine turned out to be the final stint. For reasons that remain entirely unclear, the epidemic rapidly ebbed. After treating thirty or so patients at the beginning of that last week, we closed the clinic. I embarked on my twenty-four-hour train ride back to Dacca.

The trains in Bengal were (and still are) pretty basic,

aged vehicles with hard, crowded benches. A train's "W.C." (hardly what we might think of as a lavatory) was never more than a wet and slimy little room with a hole in the floor. Two hours into the trip, I suddenly developed watery diarrhea. I thought, "I can't believe this; I've just come from treating cholera patients, and I've contracted cholera. Without any life-saving intravenous fluid or even oral rehydration solution to keep me from expiring, when the train pulls into Dacca they'll discover a dehydrated, shriveled American dead on the toilet's floor!" At every stop I purchased green coconuts and downed their contents, as good a replacement for all the fluid and electrolytes exiting at the other end as I was going to find. If I indeed had cholera, it was short-lived. By the time I arrived in Dacca my diarrhea had ceased, and I remained both lucid and alive.

Daily life for residents of Dacca was fairly languid. Phones rarely worked, local papers carried nothing but pro-government propaganda and tortured assurances that Islam really did hold women in high esteem. There was no television to speak of. The *International Herald Tribune*—an airmail subscription that cost me dearly—generally arrived a week or two after the events it described. Indeed, for the first few months we were there, it arrived in crumpled bunches, once every two or three weeks. After much frustrating enquiry, I discovered that another expatriate, who'd arrived in Dacca before me, also subscribed to the *IHT*. He had lodged a formal complaint, months before, that his copies came late, if at all, and after having obviously passed through the hands of numerous postal officials. As a result of his heated complaints to "higher authorities," all copies of the *IHT* that arrived in Dacca's central post office were immediately delivered to his address. Not wanting to disrupt this favorable resolution of his problem, he never informed the authorities of their error; so when he received both his copy and mine, he surreptitiously dropped off my (accumulated) copies whenever he happened to pass by the lab.

There was plenty of opportunity (and reason) to blissfully spend hours fantasizing about earlier visitors to the East, real and imagined: Rudyard Kipling, Somerset Maugham, famous animal tracker and storyteller Jim Corbett, and others of the British Raj. Village life encouraged it. After numerous courteous invitations from Matlab villagers that I spend an evening or two living in their village, I agreed that once the monsoon rains ended, in early October, I would return with my wife. And so I did. To the villagers' near ruination, they suggested the week following a major festival. Jill arrived appropriately encumbered in a lengthy sari, while I wore the ever-popular "pajama" pants and kurta (long white shirt). Things soon turned hilarious. Jill was quickly taken off to spend time gossiping with the women (mostly by sign language) and I became embroiled in political discussions with the men. I did worry for Jill when the time came for her to use the W.C., a flimsy wooden enclosure propped on poles strategically located 10 feet above a foul-smelling pond. You approached the enclosure by walking up two slippery, inclined logs that led from the pond's edge to the inelegantly balanced perch. All this in a full-length sari! Jill performed her ablutions with ritual splendor.

Around 5:00 in the afternoon, we were reunited and asked whether we wanted dinner. Knowing that our Bengali friends in Dacca rarely ate dinner before 9:30, we begged off, explaining, as best we could in our rudimentary Bengali, "We are happy to wait until you are ready to eat." This little act was repeated at 6:00 and again 6:30, by which time I'd wised up enough to ask, "At what time do you plan to eat?" "Oh," came the reply, "we are farmers; we ate at five o'clock, to be done before it gets dark." Chastened, and embarrassed by the extra efforts to which we had put our hosts, we sat down to a sumptuous meal, while the entire village (and then some) stood around and watched. As is village custom, many relatives had arrived the week before to attend the holiday festival. The village was prepared for the financial burden of hosting relatives during the festival, but when their guests discovered that a real Memsahib (Jill) would be coming to spend the night, they hung around an extra week to observe this unusual spectacle.

I decided I owed the village some comic relief. The next morning I volunteered to plough their field, which, if simple observation was any guide, merely meant walking behind two water buffalo as they pulled a wooden plough through the rich earth. I'd seen innumerable children do this. I handed Jill the super-8 camera to record my prowess. The village assembled, I was ceremoniously handed the buffalo reins, and quickly displayed my utter incompetence. The buffalo ignored me entirely and wandered aimlessly across the beautifully ploughed, parallel tracks from the day before. By the time we departed, the village was probably in deep financial distress, but it was also in high spirits, and our bond with those among whom I was doing fieldwork had been inestimably strengthened.

Life was simple and sweet. Until November 12, 1970.

FORGET THE JOB DESCRIPTION

Anyone who has spent a few nights in a tent during a storm can tell you: The world doesn't care all that much if you live or die.

ANTHONY DOERR

On November 12, Dacca was warm and humid, but not unbearably so. We were hosting a dinner party that evening, but we thought nothing of the darkening clouds and wind that began to build in the late afternoon. It was a typical day during the late rainy season, and it began to rain just as the guests arrived. Soon the wind and downpour seemed heavier than usual, but dinner went well, and after our guests departed Jill and I watched the wildness of nature from the protection of our covered veranda.

By early morning the storm had passed. The sky was clear blue and filled with the huge white cumulus clouds for which Dacca is famous. The storm had done little damage, at least to Dacca. Two days later, disturbing rumors, and awful photos, began to appear on local posters and in the newspapers. The storm had caused widespread death and destruction in the coastal villages to the south, bordering the Bay of Bengal.

The southern half of Bangladesh has a barely perceptible

gradient of 1 inch per mile. Much of the land on which rice is grown along the Bay of Bengal is submerged during the rainy season (June–October), none more so than the mud flats ("chars") bordering the bay. People should never have farmed these low-lying fields, let alone lived on them, but intense population pressures ensured that they did. These mud flats had received the full force of a wall of water whipped up by a cyclone in the Bay of Bengal, the same storm that had given Dacca the memorable, if brief, downpour.

Communications with the affected area were badly disrupted. A group of concerned Bengalis and expatriates collected food and relief supplies, which were loaded onto a small ferry leaving Dacca for the south. I and a few others went aboard as well, to distribute the relief supplies and lend a hand. We were soon headed south. At the end of the ferry line, our small band hitched a ride on a passing patrol boat. Its captain brought us deeper into the affected area. We finally arrived at our destination, the isolated island of Manpura, in the dead of night.

Before the cyclone, Manpura had been a cluster of villages housing about 30,000 people. We arrived to see a shore barren of everything except bloated bodies—both human and farm animals. We found a clearing along the coast, unloaded our cache, and slept among the supplies (and bodies) to prevent looting.

I'd acquired what few relief-effort skills I possessed second hand, from the reports of fellow EIS officers assisting refugees during Nigeria's Biafra conflict. Regardless of "generally accepted principles of conduct," most relief workers discover that the strongest (typically young men), not women and children, inevitably make their way to the head of the relief line. As a precautionary measure, we deputized local male villagers to assist us in organizing our efforts. We sorted our supplies, now protected by a circle of men with lathe sticks (long bamboo poles). Next, a large open area was cordoned off in hopes that supply planes might use it as a drop zone. Lastly, the local populace was lined up, women and children first, to receive our meager offerings. These were distributed without mishap.

Around midafternoon a large, lumbering C-130 cargo plane passed high overhead. To our surprise it circled back, again and again, at lower and lower altitudes. This seemed so much like a rerun of black and white World War II movies that I couldn't believe it was real. Finally, the plane began a low-level pass—at which point half a dozen villagers broke through the ranks of the deputized guards and ran to the center of the makeshift drop zone. I could only imagine the disaster if one of them tried to catch a 100-pound bag of rice dropped from 500 feet! The deputized guards rallied, the villagers were chased from the field, and sacks of rice landed without mishap.

Within half an hour we received a second surprise. A helicopter pilot had been fruitlessly searching the storm-ravaged areas for a safe place to land and deliver his load of supplies for needy survivors. Two previous attempts had been near-catastrophes; villagers swarming his helicopter had nearly been decapitated by its whirling blades (a fate subsequently suffered by an American serviceman assisting later relief efforts). The helicopter pilot had flown off and was about to give up when the cargo plane's pilot advised him that the tiny island of Manpura was well organized and had a safe and secure landing site. Being designated a "safe, organized place" meant that Manpura would eventually receive a wildly disproportionate share of all the relief delivered to the stricken region, and much of the West's media attention. All that effort was impressive for one small island—a veritable dot within the huge, decimated landscape along the Bay of Bengal.

For me the experience was transforming. Small random events—a happenstance communication between two pilots—clearly could have a major impact. On the third day of the disaster, I received an air-dropped message to return to Dacca as quickly as possible. Two days later I arrived, having, quite literally, hitched rides up-river.

I soon learned that senior staff at CRL were not happy that some of us had "abandoned" our research assignments for work in the disaster zone. But their disapproval passed quickly when the United States embassy issued an appeal for the lab's assistance. The Pakistani government had requested dozens of x-ray machines and field hospitals (stockpiled in nearby Thailand and South Vietnam). I was the only one at CRL headquarters with first-hand experience in the disaster-affected area, and I had seen little to suggest the need for either x-ray equipment or field hospitals. An earthquake can inflict severe injuries from collapsing buildings, but the cyclone's wall of water swept away everyone who was too young, too old, or too infirm to hold on to a tree. (I named the most common injury I encountered in the disaster area "cyclone syndrome"; it consisted of abrasions of the chest and inner aspects of the arms and thighs of survivors, the result of clinging tightly to a tree as the wall of water engulfed them.)

My boss, Henry Mosley, organized a rapid survey of the affected area, enlisting the help of several visiting EIS officers and two army helicopters. I was left to accompany Western cameramen, in search of stories and footage, to our Matlab facilities.

Mosley's brief survey confirmed the relatively good health of the survivors and their need for food and shelter. The field hospitals and x-ray machines that were never needed were never sent. But other relief supplies flooded into

Dacca's airport—from which only a trickle initially emerged. I was told that only the president of Pakistan could excuse donated supplies from import duties; but "the president" was "unavailable" to issue waivers, and the donors were not about to pay taxes on their donations. "Taxes on urgently needed relief donations?" "Yes." "Can't somebody other than the president exempt the supplies from import duties?" "No. If someone did, they would be held responsible for any repercussions." No action meant no fault!

And some donations were worthless: outdated drugs that could not be sold but could be "contributed" for a hefty tax break; and other drugs that often had no discernible use. I sarcastically observed that a large shipment of tranquilizers could not feed the hungry but might keep them from noticing their hunger. We received electric blankets for use in a remote tropical region that lacked electricity! These useless donations wasted everyone's time and consumed valuable shipping capacity.

Mosley's "quick and dirty" survey had proven immensely helpful in guiding immediate relief efforts, but a more detailed, extensive survey would be essential to planning the affected area's long-term reconstruction and development. Mosley assigned me this task.

What we needed was an accurate description of the present status of the population and their estimate of the losses they had suffered; exactly what a "cross-sectional" survey is designed to provide. Since we could not hope to examine the entire population, the key to accuracy would be examining and interviewing a representative sample of that population, a small fraction that would accurately reflect the situation among the population at large. The key to that would be randomly selecting the villages to be surveyed, and the families within those villages, not just the first thirty or fifty people encountered. Upon arriving at a randomly selected village, the teams made their way to the village mosque, invariably located at the heart of the village. From there they randomly chose a direction in which to walk, enrolling every family in their path.

Two small ferryboats provided headquarters and housing for me and the staff. They also towed the five speedboats we used to land study teams on remote coastal and riverside villages. Two lumbering sail-powered, wooden "country boats," carrying drums of diesel fuel for the ferries and gasoline for the speedboats, preceded us.

One of these ferries was our flagship (as it were). An enclosed area on deck served as my office and "stateroom" (with a vivid use of my imagination). Of course, my "stateroom" lacked a bed, but a narrow wooden bench, about 14 inches wide, ran along the starboard wall. Given the profusion of "wildlife" that roamed this ancient vessel each night, I decided to sleep on the bench, rather than on the floor. I'd brought along an inflatable air mattress, but it was much too wide for the narrow bench. The first few nights, I invariably awoke in free fall, headed for the floor after all. Comfort was gained, and crashes avoided, by roping both the air mattress and me to the wall that supported the bench.

Our expedition's appointed cook, haphazardly trained in both food preparation and hygiene, set up shop at the tail end of the boat. More precisely, as far back in the boat as he could go, along the starboard side, so as to have ready access to the river. This facilitated the drawing of water (including that used for drinking) and the dumping of garbage. It also provided close proximity to eliminations of another kind: the ferry's two privies (holes in the floor over which one squatted) were immediately aft of the surface on which the cook prepared our meals. Amazingly, neither I nor any member of the staff became seriously ill (no doubt thanks to the strict practice of never eating or drinking anything that was not freshly boiled). I still consider this more than a minor miracle.

In addition to the wildlife population of rodents and insects, the ferry carried a "protein supply": dozens of chickens, whose sacrifice perked up our daily rations of rice and dhal (a thin, legume gruel).

My tasks, in addition to the expected duties of dispatching the survey teams, analyzing the data collected the previous day, and choosing the next day's sample sites, included plotting our course on the river and deciding the time at which the ferries would raise anchor and depart for our next location. Being a landlubber who was using outdated colonial-era maps, I didn't always get my nautical duties right. More than once we awoke to find our ferries high and dry because I had miscalculated the timing of the tide.

I was also blissfully ignorant about the wildlife in the adjoining jungles of the Sundarbands, and the way in which some of those creatures encroached on the rivers in which we anchored—and in which I bathed each day at dusk. The villagers were wiser. On the third evening of watching me in amazement, they chastised my Bengali colleagues for letting me be so foolish. "Doesn't the 'Bora Sahib' (big shot white man) know the river is full of crocodiles?" I immediately returned to the boat. The next day I spotted my first crocodile.

The survey documented, in rigorous epidemiologic fashion, the losses of life and material, though no report could possibly capture the tragedy. By our count, at least a quarter of a million people died that dreadful night. Healthy young men fared best of all, as *only* 6 percent of them died. Among the very young and the very old, the figure approached one out of every four. Tens of thousands of livestock had been lost, along with virtually all the fishing gear and boats. Following the mourning, thoughts would need to turn to rebuilding. Livestock, boats, and gear would need to be replaced if the survivors were ever to sustain themselves and regain a semblance of their former lives.

DON'T COUNT ON THINGS STAYING THE SAME

What's important is not how to do things right,
but how to find the right things to do.

PETER DRUCKER

Nothing is stable if one takes a long enough view, but some things and some places are particularly unstable. Pakistan is one such place. What follows is a brief and selective political history of the land to which I had been sent, as it is important for understanding what we faced next.

By the early decades of the twentieth century, English rule of India was entering its endgame. The secular Congress Party had a visionary leader in Mohandas Gandhi, who was backed by prominent members of the Hindu and Muslim populations, most notably Jawaharlal Nehru and Muhammad Ali Jinnah, respectively. By 1920 Jinnah, a tweed-jacketed, pipe-smoking Muslim nationalist, had broken with the Congress Party; he eventually called for the establishment of an independent state for the subcontinent's Muslims. His initial focus was the Urdu-speaking Muslim majority concentrated in the Punjab and the rest of northwest India. Only later, when he was pushed to consider the many Muslims who lived on the other side of India, in eastern Bengal, were they included in his plans. In time, these areas became the west and east "wings" of Pakistan, divided by a roughly 1,000-mile piece of India that lay between them.

The bloodbath that accompanied the division of formerly British-ruled India into these two nations was frightful. The nation of India succeeded in becoming a multiethnic democracy, but Pakistan, particularly West Pakistan, violently rid itself of all Sikhs and Hindus. East Pakistan, which eventually became Bangladesh, was more tolerant. When we arrived in East Pakistan, Muslims made up the vast majority of the population, but Hindus still accounted for more than 10 percent, and local Hindu ceremonies were a colorful part of village life.

Although the Bengali-speaking citizens of the east wing made up a majority of Pakistan's total population, the new country's leadership was dominated by the Urdu-speaking politicians and military officers of Jinnah's home, in the west wing. Initially, Pakistan's central government declared Urdu the official language. After the inevitable language riots that followed, the law was rescinded, but the persistently west wing–centric agenda did not change. For nearly a quarter-century after the 1947 partition that created Pakistan, East and West, the country was effectively ruled by the west wing, either by an elected prime minister or by a post-coup army general. It was sometimes ruled by both, which was largely the case when we arrived in Dacca.

The real power in Pakistan in 1970 was General (and occasionally President) Agha Yahya Khan, a hunting buddy of then U.S. ambassador Joseph Farland. The civilian frontman was Zulfikar Ali Bhutto, leader of the Pakistan People's Party. Then something wholly unexpected happened.

A charismatic Bengali, Sheik Mujibur Rahman, energized the east wing's political factions and rallied them around a single party, his Awami League. If the Bengali population united behind this single leader and party, they would win a majority in the national election, dominate Parliament, and be in a position to name the prime minister. They did win—and they did name a prime minister.

Neither Yahya Khan nor Bhutto was pleased. They made it increasingly clear that they were not about to give way to an east wing, Bengali-dominated government; and they attempted to change the political rules to thwart the fact that a Bengali had won the nationwide popular vote and should, by rights, be prime minister of the entire nation, both wings.

Revolution was in the air. I couldn't drive to work, visit the market, or sit through dinner at home without being accosted by young students urging me to "support the revolution," thrusting makeshift flags of their proposed new nation, Bangladesh, into my hand. Most American expatriates were unhappy with the way West Pakistan had ridden roughshod over their east-wing brothers, but they were not necessarily in support of yet another subdivision of the subcontinent. The political kettle boiled for all to see.

Yahya Khan and Bhutto, the west wing's military-civilian complex, made several highly unpopular visits to East Pakistan. A political cartoon in the local English-language paper depicted Yahya Khan and Bhutto on the roof of Dacca's only luxury hotel (the Intercontinental) gazing out over a sea of Bangladeshi flags. The caption had Bhutto asking Yahya Khan, "Where is Pakistan?" The nationalist fever was spreading. One night, in solidarity with student urging, we flew a student-sewn version of the proposed new flag from our own roof.

At 1:30 in the morning, March 26, 1971, Jill and I awoke. At first we heard only the drone of our bedroom air conditioners. But within a few moments we made out soft thudding sounds in the background. Jill asked me what I thought they might be. I suggested thunder. No, they were too regular. "Ah," I responded, "Yahya Khan and Bhutto are departing for the west wing, and receiving a twenty-one-gun salute."

Unconvinced, she asked, "Why are they leaving in the middle of the night?"

I shrugged off the sleep and said, "They are sneaking out of town."

"If they are sneaking out of town," she continued, "why are they receiving a twenty-one-gun salute?"

When the force of Jill's logic struck home we bounded from bed and ran up to the roof. Jon and Candy Rohde were seated on their roof, ten feet away. They motioned to long lines of tanks streaming from the cantonment, just up the road. Old Dacca, several miles away, was ablaze.

Jon looked over and said, "It's about time you guys got up. We've been pounding on your doors and windows. We had our cook take that damned flag down from your roof."

During the next twenty-four hours, we knew little about what was happening. Martial law and a curfew were in effect and rumors swirled about. Our suburban neighborhood was untouched and eerily quiet. Pakistani television reported that nothing had happened; and if by chance it had, "everything was back to normal." The scenes they showed of Dacca—shuttered homes and markets, not a single vehicle of any sort moving downtown—looked anything but normal.

When we moved to Dacca, U.S. government regulations required us to bring our existing cars. Jill and I possessed what was perhaps the most noticeable vehicle on all of the Indian subcontinent, a canary yellow Dodge Dart convertible. On the second day after the coup we were given permission to travel around town, though few people did. John Stoeckel, a demographer and colleague at the laboratory (with an equally young infant at home and equal curiosity), suggested that he and I drive around town to see what might have happened. In the canary yellow car, we headed straight for the racecourse, a downtown remnant of the old Raj and longtime home to a small, displaced Hindu community. The sight that awaited us was appalling: bloodied bodies of men, women, and children, and walls pock-marked from machine gun fire. We decided we'd seen enough and returned home, dispirited and outraged.

That evening Pakistani TV again announced that everything had returned to normal, and they backed that claim with repeated footage of my yellow Dodge Dart trolling around Dacca.

To our embarrassment and dismay, nearly all Bengalis insisted, "America will not stand for this trampling on our democracy and human rights." We Americans sadly knew otherwise.

Bengali politicians and intellectuals feared for their lives. Like other expatriates, we hid prominent Bengalis in our home. I was able to transport some of them, hidden in the trunk of our car, to the relative safety of the rural countryside. From there, most made their way across the border to India.

It may seem odd, but we were not really frightened. We had come to believe (rightly or wrongly) that white Westerners, Bora Sahibs, still enjoyed the special status they'd acquired during the British Raj. Whenever I encountered a roadblock manned by towering paramilitary Northwest Frontier militia, I'd yell out that I was an American doctor. They would simply get out of the way.

Troops from West Pakistan were continuously flown into the east wing on Pakistan Airlines planes. Because India prohibited over-flights of its territory and threatened to conduct anti-aircraft rocket "practice," the planes had to refuel in Sri Lanka (formerly Ceylon). For pure political theater, nothing surpassed the supposed civilian nature of these flights. On landing at Dacca's airport, the "civilian" passengers all dressed in jackets and ties, descended from the planes, formed tight formations, and marched smartly off the field. In an hour the civilian clothes were traded for military fatigues.

Western nations began evacuating their staff and dependents, but the United States continued to suggest that nothing was amiss. Henry Kissinger, then U.S. secretary of state and master of realpolitick, later explained that America had "tilted towards Pakistan."

The Stoeckel family and ours decided to send our servants home to the comparative safety of the countryside. The Stoeckels then moved in with us, and we consolidated our essentials. John and I made an oath that we'd not leave a drop of liquor behind for the Pakistani troops!

Each evening John and I sat on the veranda, making steady progress on our pledge, while watching lightning mixed with the flashes and sounds of machine guns. Every hour on the hour, Jill and Marsha would join us around the shortwave radio for news from the BBC. Minutes before the hourly tolling of Big Ben (that normally preceded the news), we listened as the voice on the radio gravely announced: "This is a special message for Her Majesty's subjects in East Pakistan. Make your way as soon as possible to Chittagong port, where Her Majesty has sent a ship to evacuate you. You will, of course, be expected to reimburse Her Majesty's government upon landing at Southampton." To use an old cliché, you can't make this stuff up.

John and I sometimes took our special status as Bora Sahibs to naïve and dangerous lengths. One evening we discovered that, when moving their supplies into our house, we had salvaged their instant pizza mix but not the accompanying sauce. Despite the curfew and distant machine gun fire, we sneaked three blocks to their old house to retrieve it. Pizza never tasted so good.

By early April, most Westerners, excepting Americans, had been evacuated. Most American expatriates were outraged at our government's complicity. We demanded a meeting with our consul general, Archer Blood, the highest-ranking American official in East Pakistan. He was sympathetic, and he had the power to order our evacuation (this was a political gesture on our part—few of us actually felt endangered). And so he did. His immediate superior, the U.S. ambassador to Pakistan and hunting buddy of Yahya Khan, who was headquartered in West Pakistan, was less than fully supportive; but the CG, being on site, had the final word. This action by Archer Blood was not, I later learned, without repercussions to his career; in his book *The Cruel Birth of Bangladesh* he recounts how he was punished for agreeing to our evacuation.

During the year we had been in Dacca, the circumstances in which we found ourselves had changed greatly.

FOLLOW MOST, BUT NOT ALL, OF THE RULES

If there's a fork in the road, take it.

YOGI BERRA

W hat might seem to some an insignificant issue loomed large at this moment. In the hastily arranged evacuation, we learned, dogs were not allowed to accompany evacuees. What were we to do with Bacchus, our six-year-old Cairn terrier? To leave him behind meant certain agony—his and ours. Dogs were not well treated by the Muslim population, by whom they are considered unclean. In addition, most of the residents of East Pakistan were poor and frightened. He'd become an abused, mangy "pye dog," if he survived at all. We couldn't bear the thought.

I sent Jill and Charles upstairs to a bedroom while I attempted to give Bacchus a lethal injection of lidocain to stop his heart. I was feeling dreadful and consequently I bungled the execution. Bacchus pulled his paw away in fright, sensing my emotional state. Poor Bacchus whimpered uncontrollably. Half anesthetized, he dragged his way across the hall. Moving after him I glanced up, to discover Jill and Charles staring down from the second floor balcony in horror. I was in absolute misery, and I lost my nerve. I found Jon Rohde at home, next door, and begged him to do the deed. We buried Bacchus in a secluded part of our garden. Jon and Candy's cat fared better. After he was anesthetized, Candy "wore" him, as a stole, aboard the evacuation flight.

It took six flights to evacuate all of the Americans. A group of us volunteered for the last flight out, on April 6, because we planned to stage a protest once the plane landed in Sri Lanka to refuel. If we were on an earlier flight, doing so might endanger the lives of Americans still in East Pakistan. Someone clearly spilled the beans about our plans. Our passports were confiscated as we boarded the evacuation flight and the plane never opened its doors during refueling in Sri Lanka.

The U.S. government (always "tilting towards Pakistan") subsidized the cost of flying Pakistan's troops from the west wing to the east wing, by paying Pakistan to evacuate us in the otherwise empty planes flying in the opposite direction. We were outraged. It meant a much longer flight than the originally planned trip to Bangkok (using U.S. Air Force planes), and worse, we were being sent to the west wing, the "enemy" (in our view). We protested loudly upon landing in Karachi, so the next day we were flown, by chartered Pan Am 707, to Tehran (which shows just how much has changed—Tehran was then a safe haven for Americans!).

As the plane took off from Karachi headed to Iran, the pilot said, "Welcome home to America." There was a loud cheer—and then handkerchiefs and sobs. Few of us had recognized just how much strain we'd been under until it was suddenly lifted. Bright lights and movie cameras from all the major television networks greeted our arrival in Tehran. Candy Rohde was captured on the newsreels descending the jetway elegantly attired in her (once again anesthetized) cat stole.

Jill's parents and mine saw us deplane on the evening news. When they called the embassy the next day to check on our well-being and chat, they were informed that "Dr. Sommer and his family have apparently gone off to a remote area to attend a camel market." Indeed we had, and it was a twenty-hour train ride away. We stayed at a local hotel overnight and took a taxi to the barren plain on which the monthly market was held. There were no camels, but an ancient, elaborately turbaned trader was sitting cross-legged beside six lovely pieces of tribal jewelry. One silver pendant, with large rough-cut stones, caught Jill's eye. Having learned to be a canny bargainer, she asked what I thought it was worth. I asked her how much she was prepared to spend. We agreed our limit was $5. Jill asked his price. He replied, "75 cents." Jill bargained, as was the custom. He wouldn't budge. She walked away—and never bought it!

"Why not?" I asked her.

"Because he wouldn't bargain," she replied.

I said, "So what? He wants less than a fifth of what we were prepared to pay."

My by-then seasoned-traveler wife said, "Because he is treating us like tourists; if I were a local he would have bargained."

I remember thinking, someone may have lost a kingdom for lack of a horse, but we lost a beautiful silver pendant for what was probably an honest opening bid.

Because I was scheduled to deliver a research paper at the Centers for Disease Control, we were one of the first of our Dacca crowd to return to the States. Immediately upon landing at Kennedy Airport I called the Cholera Research Laboratory's administrator at NIH to report my return. I was astonished when she informed me that I was now stationed in Tehran and should return there as soon as my meeting was over. We were stunned but pleased. We had already signed up for an extra year overseas and had worried we would be kept stateside.

The CRL administrator soon rethought the situation, however. The next group of colleagues to arrive from Tehran was ordered to remain in the United States, because it seemed unlikely that the CRL would resume operations in East Pakistan anytime soon.

I called my boss (the new EIS director) at CDC, Phil Brachman, for advice.

"What should we do?" I asked.

"What do you want to do?" he replied.

"Go back overseas; I didn't sign up for an extra year to spend it in Atlanta." I said.

He advised, "Then go. Just don't contact anyone until you have left the U.S."

So we went underground. Other than Phil and our parents, no one knew our plans. We got as far as San Francisco undetected. At airport baggage collection I heard an ominous refrain:

"Would Dr. Sommer please contact the operator? Dr. Alfred Sommer."

If ever I suffered a moment of moral indecision, this was it. Who could want me, or know where I was? If we ignored the call we were home free. But it might also be an emergency. Besides, I was an officer in the United States Public Health Service (a lieutenant commander, no less); if it was an order, it was my duty to receive it, however reluctantly.

It turned out to be the head of the Special Pathogens Branch of the CDC. He'd learned of our predicament and wanted to know whether I'd be willing to run a leprosy vaccine trial in Ethiopia, which was in need of a field epidemiologist.

I remember saying, "I've never been to Ethiopia."

He replied, "Great. We'll keep in touch."

We took the long way back to Tehran, stopping in Bali, Singapore, Burma (also called Myanmar), and Nepal (where a team from the U.S. Agency for International Development [USAID] asked us to stay and work).

We'd always wanted to visit Burma, but until that month tourism stays had been limited to twenty-four hours. Suddenly Burma had begun issuing visas good for a week. We jumped at the chance. The country had long been "closed" by order of a military junta. Once known as the rice bowl of Asia, Burma had become deeply impoverished (as it remains today). Its official currency, the khat, was worth only one-tenth the official rate of exchange. Imprudently, I exchanged US$300 under a railway bridge in Singapore for 14,000 khat, theoretically enough to see us through the week. Oddly, it was illegal to import Burmese currency into Burma, so I secreted the wad in my shoes, adding just under an inch to my height.

Rangoon was dreadfully rundown; not just poor, but outright shabby. Most cars were vintage 1930s Plymouths and Chevrolets. It was hot and humid, the monsoon season, made all the more miserable by swarms of locusts.

Rangoon was also palpably scary. Since I traveled on an official government employee passport, I checked in at the American embassy upon arrival. Everyone spoke in a whisper for fear of being overheard. We soon suspected that every emaciated bicycle-rickshaw driver wore a badge under his threadbare T-shirt. With so many khats in hand, we opted to stay at the once opulent Strand Hotel.

We were shown to an enormous room by a uniformed bellhop who whispered, "Since the British left, things have gone terribly downhill." We couldn't help but suspect that he was an *agent provocateur*, but in all likelihood he was probably telling us how he felt. The Strand predated air conditioning and was intent on preserving its traditions: long sleeves and tie were required of gentlemen for afternoon tea in the lounge and dinner in the dining room, regardless of the monsoon heat and humidity.

Although we had booked three nights, I was asked, the next morning, to pay for the past night's room and dinner. This "pay as you go" plan was in place for a reason. The published rate, US$250 a night, was—precisely the expected payment. The hotel did not accept khat! We decided it surely wasn't worth the price, and we headed for the local YMCA, where we could stay at roughly 50 cents a night. It was barely worth that, even after we'd spent an extra 50 cents to have them scrub the room and provide us with clean towels and sheets.

These complaints aside, Burma and the Burmese were wonderful. Unwilling to be jailed for smuggling 10,000 remaining khats *out* of the country, we blew them on ancient Buddhist manuscripts and a beautifully wrought silver bowl we found at Rangoon's main market. Jill also acquired amebic dysentery, which fortunately wouldn't raise its ugly head until a month later, when we were back in Tehran, where colleagues at the American military hospital were able to deal with it. This was the most serious tropical disease any member of our family acquired in our many years of living and traveling overseas.

From Burma we headed to Nepal, where I spent a month assisting the health unit at USAID. Just as I was about to accept their offer of full-time employment in Nepal, I received a telex message ordering our return to Tehran in preparation for reassignment to the leprosy trial in Ethiopia. The timing actually seemed perfect. We had enjoyed our stay in Nepal, but the monsoons were beginning, making further trekking out of the question. And we'd never been to Africa.

We arrived back in Tehran to discover the Ethiopian position had fallen through, because the U.S. government wouldn't assign a federal employee to a Norwegian-funded project. We decided it was probably time to return to the States, especially as Jill was now five months pregnant with our second child. But first we decided to see a bit of East Africa. Once we had two children, we reasoned, overseas travel would prove too difficult. We later completely abandoned that pessimistic view.

I'd saved an article from the *International Herald Tribune* extolling the virtues of camping through East Africa's game parks. At the time no one knew if it was safe to take anti-malaria drugs during pregnancy. Not to chance it, we decided that Jill wouldn't; instead she would wear long sleeves and slacks, liberally smear herself with insect repellent (which might, in retrospect, have been more toxic than the drugs), and we'd spray our sleeping quarters.

We had put up at Kenya's once-proud Brunner Hotel (long since shuttered). Before going to bed we carefully scanned the walls and ceiling for telltale spots of smeared blood and small, flittering shadows of mosquitoes. All seemed to be in order, and we felt fairly safe from the threat of malaria. Out went the lights. Within minutes we heard that distinctive buzz. Lights on, swatter out. We killed two mosquitoes and tried to go back to sleep. It was clear we would never relax unless Jill took malaria prophylaxis. And so she did; our daughter, Marni, turned out fine.

We rented a Peugeot 405 (the perennial Trans-Africa Rally winner) from Hertz, and all the camping gear we needed from Hamid's Camping and Safari Supplies. These would be the most eventful two weeks we'd ever spend camping. Nearly four decades later it's quite clear that this expedition was sheer lunacy born of overwhelming naïveté.

Our trip was off-season, and so we nearly always had the camp grounds to ourselves. At our first stop, Amboseli National Park, our tent faced a huge expanse of savannah.

The foreground was filled with zebra, giraffe, and wilde-beest. Mount Kenya loomed behind. Mindful of the wildlife, we stayed in the car. As they seemed placid enough, how-ever, we turned the car off and wandered about. Near dusk we returned to our campsite, only to discover that the car wouldn't start. The battery was dead, probably, I deduced, from a faulty alternator. It was now getting dark. I decided I'd best get word to Hertz, if possible, and so I left Charles and Jill at the tent with a lantern burning and hiked towards a lodge we had passed two miles up the road. About half-way there, as I emerged from the bush, I found myself fac-ing a herd of Cape buffalo. I froze, unable to decide if this was simply bad or truly terrible. I knew that Cape buffalo are among the meanest creatures on earth; I just hadn't ex-pected to meet any, let alone that many.

I was saved (quite likely in a literal sense) by the lights of an oncoming vehicle. It was a game warden heading home for dinner at the lodge. He stopped for me but was none too pleased and thoroughly admonished me. I contacted Hertz on the lodge's radio. The ranger then gave me a second lec-ture, and a ride back to the tent. Our car was replaced the following day.

We returned to Atlanta after our explorations and moved into a lovely little house that friends had rented for us. I spent the next few months analyzing data from the cyclone survey, preparing the study report for publication, and mak-ing plans to return to Dacca, once the war was won, to as-sist in relief and rehabilitation. Bangladesh was all the rage in those days (the start of feel-good celebrity events, like the Concert for Bangladesh), and my heart was with the people there.

Pakistan's civil war came to an abrupt end when In-dia entered on the side of Bangladesh. Soon afterward, the United Nations initiated relief efforts under the acronym

UNROD (United Nations Relief Operations Dacca). I was quick to offer up plans for a postwar survey to assess national losses and guide relief efforts. The United States, having favored Pakistan, had no interest in sending me to assist; and the new consul general (America was not about to bless the new nation with an ambassador) did not want to incur the potential political risks associated with having American officials wandering about the countryside.

Within weeks it became apparent that Bangladesh was in the early stages of a potentially massive smallpox epidemic. Having broken out in the refugee camps in India, the disease was now being spread by the millions of people migrating back home. UNROD appealed to the World Health Organization for assistance and I was asked by CDC to be part of a three-person international team being assembled to initiate smallpox control measures. It was again time to pack.

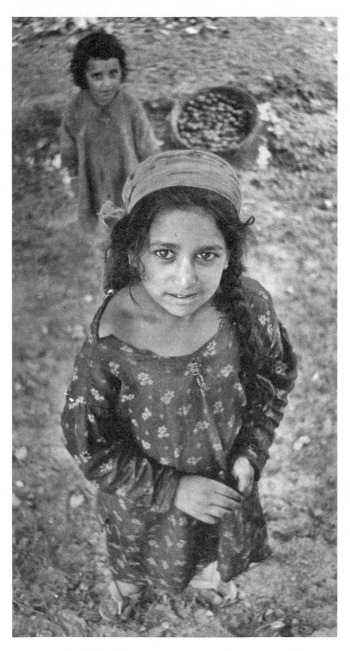

A young girl and her sibling at a rural camel market in northwest Iran. We encountered them after our evacuation to Iran following the onset of civil war in 1971 in East Pakistan.

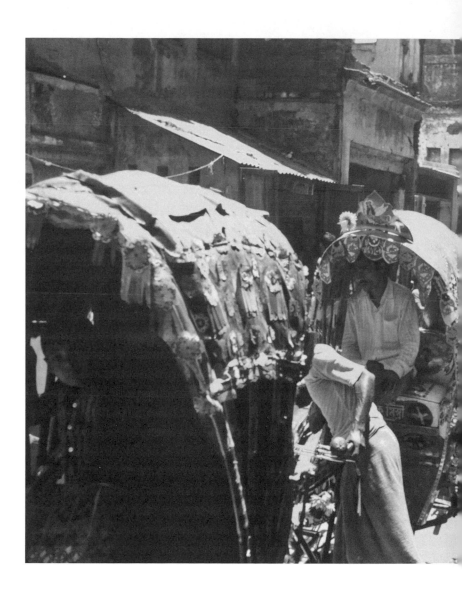

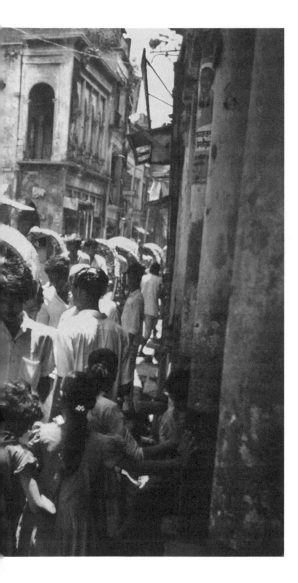

The crowded warrens of Old Dacca, where Jill and I got lost (and much delayed) in route to a formal dinner with Bangladesh's first president, Abu Sayeed Chowdhury, at his official residence. It was three days before we would leave the country for the last time, after initiating smallpox control efforts and a postwar survey, in the spring of 1972.

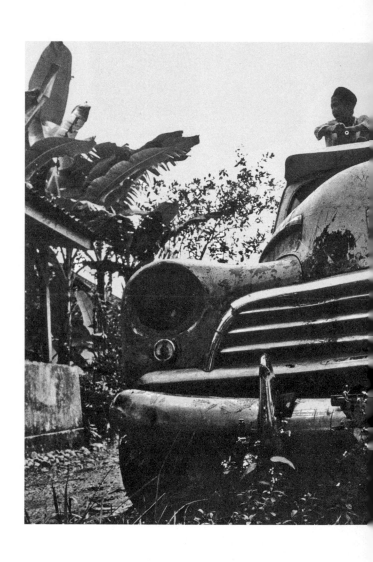

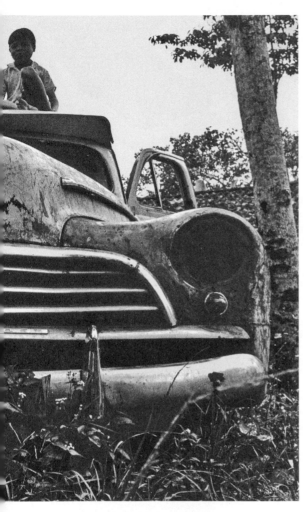

An abandoned, stripped American car from the 1940s, still useful as a playground in 1976. It was at the end of a rural village road in Indonesia. My colleague Pak Tarwotjo memorably noted, "It's forty years old and still on the road."

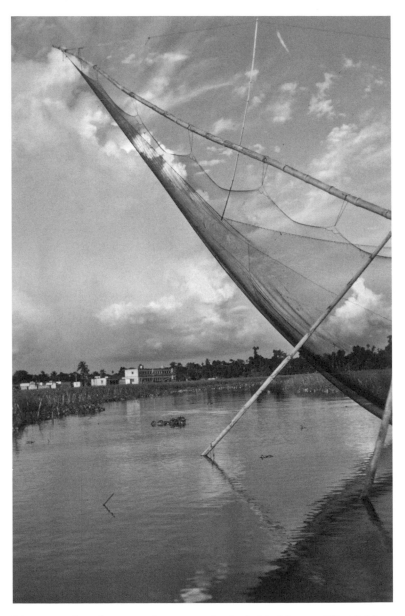

Rivers were the only means of transportation in the Matlab area of East Pakistan in the 1970s. We saw giant fishing nets, like the one shown in the foreground in its raised position, at regular intervals as we traveled to the Matlab Cholera Hospital, our central research and treatment facility, seen here in the background.

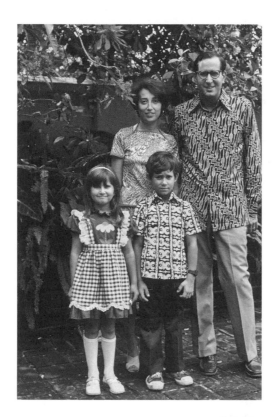

The Sommer family, Marni, Jill, Charles, and Al, in the garden behind our home on Jalan Setia Budhi, Bandung, Indonesia, in 1976. Charles and I are wearing Batik shirts, traditional in Indonesia.

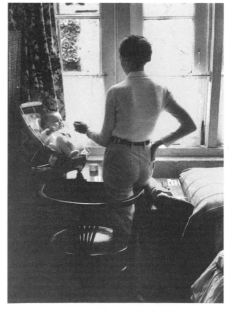

Jill feeding Marni, then four months old, during our temporary return to the former East Pakistan, newly independent and named Bangladesh, in 1972.

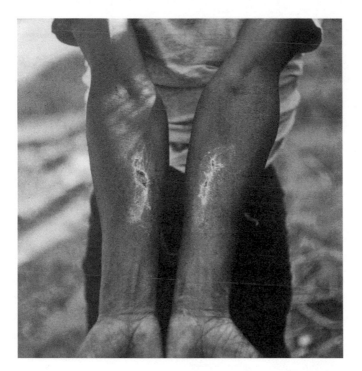

The most common injuries we encountered during a survey of the
cyclone destruction along the Bay of Bengal in late 1970 were abrasions on the inner arms and thighs and on the chest. They were
caused by holding tightly to trees as the 100-foot wave of water
rushed by. The name I gave this set of clinical signs was "cyclone
syndrome."

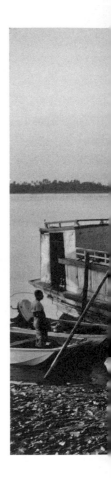

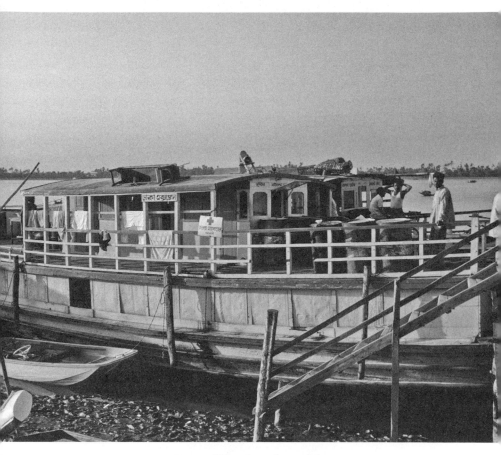

Two small ferryboats housed the crew, our survey teams, our cooking facilities, and our "protein supplies" (live chickens). We towed five speed boats (*three seen at left*) to reach the cyclone-devastated villages along the Bay of Bengal. One ferry served as my "command ship." It was off this boat, after what turned out to be my last day of bathing in the river at dusk, that I saw my first crocodile.

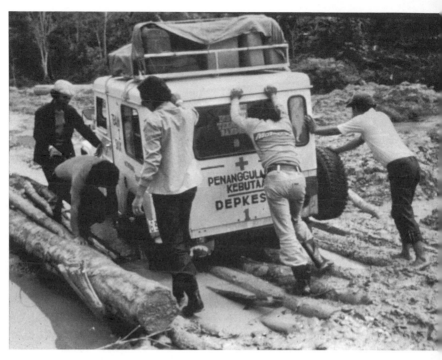

Conducting field studies and randomized village-based trials of vitamin A supplementation meant first getting to the villages. The roads were often only mud ditches, sometimes further obstructed by fallen trees. In this photo, we are pushing our jeep in Aceh Province, Sumatra, Indonesia, in 1983.

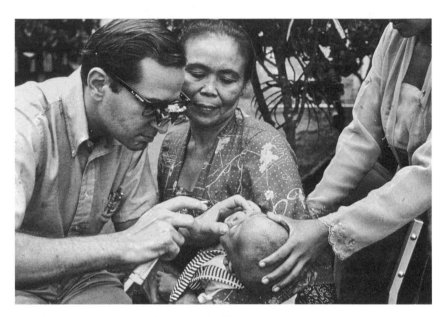

Examining an Indonesian child with night blindness and other evidence of xerophthalmia, the ocular manifestations of vitamin A deficiency, at the Cicendo Eye Hospital, in Bandung, Indonesia, in 1976.

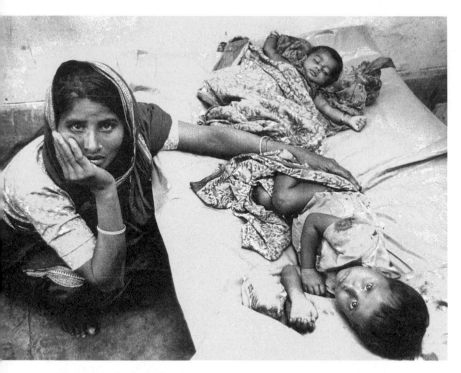

A worried mother and two young children with cholera on a typical cholera cot at the Cholera Research Laboratory's research and treatment hospital in Dacca in 1971.

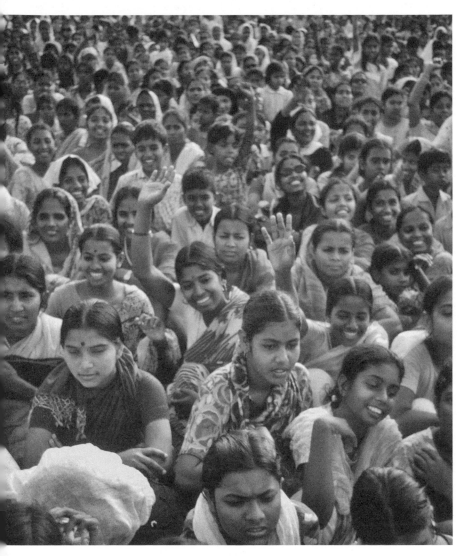

Part of a crowd who assembled to welcome Bangladesh's founding prime minister, Sheik Mujibur Rahman, shortly after the end of the War of Liberation and his release from a Pakistani prison in 1972. I used fake media credentials to get to the front of the stadium in which the rally took place.

COLLECT GOOD DATA—
Even If You Don't Yet Know
What Important Questions
They May Answer

Results are obtained by exploiting opportunities.

PETER DRUCKER

I knew almost nothing about smallpox, but I did know the countryside of what was now Bangladesh. Stan Foster, a colleague on the team, had spent seven years working on smallpox in Nigeria, and he knew everything there was to know about smallpox, but he had no experience in Asia. On the flight to Dacca, we began educating each other.

Stan and I had an important job and were given all the support available, but that support was very limited. The minister of health's nephew was appointed director of Bangladesh's Smallpox Eradication Program. He was about my age, had received his medical education in Bangladesh and Lebanon, and spoke fluent English. One of the first things I noticed about him was his love of his title, his authority, and his big desk. The day we arrived was his second day on the job. I suggested that we visit the infectious disease hospital outside Dacca to get some sense of the disease we were dealing with and the state of the epidemic. After we parked in front of the large, isolated building, I discovered that he had no intention of going inside.

Nothing I said could persuade him to enter the building. The reason suddenly dawned on me. Bangladesh's director of smallpox eradication had never been vaccinated against smallpox! This was a bad omen, both regarding the leadership of the program and the local opinion about vaccinations. If the director of the program, a well-trained physician, was still unvaccinated, it was highly unlikely that the many friends and relatives visiting patients in the hospital were vaccinated.

A quick survey confirmed that many of the visitors lacked the easily recognized vaccination scar. In essence, the hospital was serving as a central repository and distribution center of infection. Those visiting their loved ones were contracting the disease and spreading it to their families and friends back home. My first useful act was to station guards at the hospital's door to vaccinate everyone before they entered.

The most intense focus of infection at that moment was in Khulna District, a coastal region in the south of the country. It became my task to organize local control efforts. It soon became apparent that we were dealing with two distinct outbreaks: a generalized epidemic moving inexorably through the town of Khulna, the provincial capital, and, some miles away in the countryside, a second epidemic within a densely inhabited refugee camp. These were "reverse" refugees, a group of Urdhu speakers who had come to East Pakistan from Bihar at the time of original partition. They had never assimilated into the local, Bengali culture and were considered by many Bangladeshis to have been collaborators in the West Pakistani occupation.

Epidemic-control programs depend upon zeal and common sense. Common sense told me that the outbreak in Khulna City could be stopped by the new "surveillance and containment" strategy: find new cases and vaccinate all their potential contacts. Obsessed with collecting data, I designed surveillance forms and insisted that the field workers keep careful notes on all cases, family members, and other contacts. These data enabled us to demonstrate, for the first time in a rigorous fashion, that surveillance and containment actually worked. Wherever we initiated vaccination efforts, the epidemic stopped within days.

The situation in the towns was bad enough, but the crowded refugee camp was another matter altogether. The people were desperately poor and entirely dependent on relief rations. They lived in thin, small tents that were occupied by often large, over-extended families. The sick and dying were everywhere, and the scene was nothing less than apocalyptic. Because everyone had potential contact with an infected person, the only sensible approach seemed to be to vaccinate everyone. Time was absolutely of the essence. We began, vaccinating more than 2,000 people a day. Within two weeks we had vaccinated 31,000 people, at least 75 percent of the camp's inhabitants.

Unfortunately, not everyone wanted our help; a substantial proportion of the population was suspicious of vaccination. They remained a threat to themselves and to the larger community. We acted on the moment with proselytizing zeal. As others have reported doing under similar circumstances, we coerced the population in ways that might not be condoned today. I refused to issue food rations to anyone who had not been vaccinated. That turned the tide. It was, no doubt, an arrogant decision, but one I have never regretted.

That refugee camp taught me a lesson about the ingenuity (and despair) of people who are powerless and dependent upon others for survival. I awoke early one morning, about 4:00 a.m., too restless to sleep. I was pretty much alone in a Dhak bungalow a mile or so from the camp. As I walked down the country path I became aware of a line of wispy, shrouded figures moving, some distance away, through the early morning fog. I couldn't imagine what anyone (besides me) would be doing up at that hour. I soon found out: it was a procession of refugees from the camp carrying their dead to the cemetery. Why bury the dead at such an hour? To hide the fact that they had died and thereby to retain their ration cards. This suggested a useful surveillance strategy: cemetery burials as a way to monitor smallpox epidemics and gauge the effectiveness of control efforts. A comparison between registered burials and the progress of the epidemic as reported in data collected by the vaccination teams proved its value. This tactic is similar to the tracking of pharmacy purchases and hospitalizations used by today's epidemilogists to identify and follow early outbreaks of infectious diseases.

Another important insight would emerge from that smallpox control effort in Khulna—but its practical impact would not be felt until three decades later. The anthrax attacks in the United States following 9/11 led to considerable hysteria over the imminent risk of more widespread bioterrorist attacks. The idea took hold that suicide terrorists would infect themselves from clandestinely hoarded stores of smallpox virus and cause massive outbreaks—perhaps by riding the New York subways. President Bush ordered the immediate vaccination of millions of first responders, which might itself have been a catastrophe. The vaccine that had eradicated naturally occurring cases of smallpox around the world was actually quite primitive; massive vaccination with it would undoubtedly maim or kill many with poor immune responses, and the number of people with poor immunity had grown dramatically with the widespread use of cancer chemotherapy and the advent of HIV. But data from that long ago smallpox control effort in Bangladesh, published at the same time as the cemetery surveillance paper, demonstrated that vaccination as late as six days after initial infection provided complete protection from the disease. Anthony Fauci, director of the National Institute of Allergy and Infectious Disease, opened a one-day meeting at the Institute of Medicine to review the president's policy. Tony's first chart came from that second, thirty-year-old paper from Bangladesh. Because public health officials could wait nearly a week to vaccinate anyone who might have been exposed to a real case of smallpox, it made more sense to stock the vaccine at convenient locations, should it ever be needed, rather than waste money and lives vaccinating millions of people against something that might never happen.

REMEMBER YOUR HUMANITY

Living a successful and satisfying life depends in great
measure on early distinguishing between things which
matter much and things which matter little.

E. V. MCCOLLUM

||||||||||||||||||||||||||||||||||||||||||||||||||||||||||||||||||||||||||||||||||||||||||||||||||||||||||||||||||||||||||||||

S everal days before we had been evacuated from Dacca
during the civil war (or, to the Bangladeshis, the War
of Liberation), a prominent Bengali had come to our home.
He had written two dozen names on a tiny piece of paper; all
were prominent Bengali intellectuals and politicians who'd
been murdered by the occupying Pakistani army. He asked
that I deliver the list to a particular Bengali barrister in London. Of course, I said I would.

I knew that upon boarding the evacuation flights we
would be searched, and any intelligence would be confiscated. I therefore concealed the slip of paper inside a slit
I made in my trouser belt. I felt like an actor in a grade B
WWII movie, but I knew that this was not a laughing matter. My visitor had risked his life by preparing and delivering
the list.

After the few days in Iran we boarded our flight to
London in route back to the United States. In London, we
stayed overnight at Green's Hotel. I telephoned a number I

had been given and late that afternoon was visited by the barrister in question. He brought along an impressive, older Bengali gentleman, Abu Sayeed Chowdhury. I soon learned that I was in the presence of the highly respected chief justice of the Pakistani Supreme Court. In a quirk of irony, the day the Pakistan army struck Dacca, the chief justice had been out of the country, representing Pakistan at an international conference on human rights. He was now the roving ambassador for the nascent nation of his birth, Bangladesh. We spoke in hushed tones in a room at the rear of the hotel's lobby. It had the eerie feeling of a scene from *Casablanca*.

A mere sixteen months later, Abu Sayeed Chowdhury became the first president of Bangladesh. We were in Bangladesh because of the smallpox epidemic and just a few days from returning to the States for good. I sent a note to President Chowdhury, asking if by chance Jill and I might briefly congratulate him in person on the war's outcome. I doubted he would even remember me. To my amazement, a beribboned colonel appeared at my office that same afternoon, bearing a gold-engraved invitation to attend dinner at the Presidential Palace the next evening. Jill and I were dumbfounded. What does one wear to the Presidential Palace? Surely something more formal than my khaki field clothes and Jill's cotton shift and slacks. We convinced ourselves it would be a big party; we could sneak in, pay our respects, and be gone before anyone noticed. We drove to the palace in our only means of transport: my white, topless "smallpox jeep." In route I got hopelessly lost in Old Dacca; we arrived at the gates of the palace twenty minutes late. The grounds were huge—and dark. We saw very few cars (certainly too few for the big party we had imagined).

Armed soldiers blocked our path. I told them we had been invited to dinner by the president. Not unreasonably, given our dress and mode of transport, they didn't believe us.

They called the palace and announced, "There is a Doctor Sommer who claims to have been invited to dinner with the president . . . [pause] . . . Yes, I see. Right away."

The guard turned to me. "You're late; the president is waiting for you."

And so he was, on the steps to the palace, formally attired. We discovered this was his first official reception for the ambassadors of the major Western nations: France, Germany, England, and, of course, the United States. He led us through a huge, chandeliered hall to a small, intimate sitting room where all the ambassadors and their wives were waiting in formal attire. We were more than a bit abashed by how inappropriately attired we were.

President Chowdhury clearly remembered our brief, previous encounter. He escorted Jill and me into the sitting room, arms around our shoulders, and announced to the gathering, "These two young Americans are heroes of our revolution." The new American consul general, who had done everything he could to keep me out of the country (he feared rumors of CIA work if an American was spending his time in the field), turned ashen. A professional, he quickly recovered, jumped to his feet, and, hand extended, exclaimed, "Dr. Sommer, how good to see you."

The dinner table was grand. We were prominently seated on either side of the president. Toward the end of dinner, I saw the French ambassador slip the place card with the presidential seal and his own name in gold lettering into his pocket. I had been eyeing the card all night and now felt the courage to snitch mine as well. That card was a memento and a symbol. I wasn't much of a hero; the man who gave me the list was, but I helped when I could. It's a tricky thing working in a foreign land, because it is always easy to mistakenly do something that is culturally inappropriate. But you will generally not go wrong by doing the "right" thing.

LESSON **8**

USE DATA TO SET POLICY

Research is like peeling an onion. You're ignorant at the start, you take off more layers, and you find it more and more concentrated; a denser and denser node of ignorance. And all the time you're weeping about how much it costs to get there.

FRANCIS D. MOORE

‖‖‖

Enlistment in the Epidemic Intelligence Service and my experience in Bangladesh transformed my interests and the trajectory of my career. Having experienced the thrill of discovery and the immense, immediate impact data could have on the health and well-being of whole populations, I delayed my ophthalmology residency to become formally trained in epidemiology. As a result, I began my ophthalmology training with an entirely different mindset from that of my peers. Fortunately my ophthalmology chief, Edward Maumenee, the longtime professor and director of the Wilmer Eye Institute at Johns Hopkins Hospital, was more than tolerant.

One day, relatively early in my training, Maumenee casually remarked, "Al, wasn't that a great article about the relationship between diabetes and mortality in this month's *American Journal of Ophthalmology*?" In my (commonly) unsubtle fashion, I replied, "No, it was pretty dumb. The study was full of biases, poorly analyzed, and inappropri-

51

ately interpreted. In fact most ophthalmic clinical research is poorly done, because most clinical researchers have never learned basic epidemiology." Ed was a generous and supportive mentor. "That's very interesting, Al; you should write an editorial on the subject." All I could think was, "Sure, I've just begun my ophthalmology training and I'm about to tell the ophthalmology world that they do lousy research. Besides, who has the time?"

Some mentors are good at motivating you; some are brilliant! Three days later I received a letter from Frank Newall, longstanding editor of the *AJO*. "Dear Dr. Sommer, Professor Maumenee has told me about the brilliant editorial you have written. I look forward to receiving it within the week." I spent the next five days writing a "brilliant editorial," replete with graphic illustrations culled from the publications of highly respected "giants" in the field (I didn't consider it sporting to gore only undistinguished oxen). The editorial was well received, and those I "gored" graciously forgave my youthful indiscretion.

By July 1976 I had completed my epidemiology and clinical training and had come to three realizations: (1) I was one of the few ophthalmologists trained in epidemiology; (2) I had extensive experience working in underdeveloped nations, and I loved it; and (3) I could make a bigger difference using my interests and skill set working on problems in the developing world than by pursuing a traditional academic path. It was therefore no surprise that, late that summer, we found ourselves settled in Indonesia.

One night, while supervising teams conducting a countrywide survey of vitamin A deficiency and its blinding complication, xerophthalmia, I was put up at a guest house in Surabaya that belonged to the university's eye hospital. This house was a local shrine of sorts. It had been the home of Johanna Ten Doeschatte, a devoted Dutch ophthalmologist who had spent most of her professional career working at the hospital and training its young Indonesian ophthalmologists.

I awoke at one o'clock in morning having dreamt that a huge cockroach was sitting on my face. (Despite having lived in many places where cockroaches abounded, I still detested them.) It turned out that my nightmare was true: a huge cockroach *was* sitting on my face. Dozens more were scrimmaging in the center of the floor. I went berserk, squashed all I could reach with the sole of my shoe, and then huddled, pulse racing, in the center of the bed. There was absolutely no chance I would fall back to sleep. Instead, I prepared the outline for a simple book on epidemiologic and statistical principles, to help ophthalmologists conduct more meaningful clinical research. This book, I thought, would be my contribution to correcting the unhappy state of affairs I had described in my "brilliant" editorial.

I envisioned a book that would be clear, crisp, brief, and cheap; something the average ophthalmologist could master in a single evening. To keep ophthalmologists' interest, every principle would be illustrated by examples drawn from the ophthalmic literature. I completed the manuscript over the course of the next month.

Ron Michaels, my former chief resident, encouraged me to send my manuscript to a major medical publishing house; he was certain they'd be interested. I did; they weren't, at least not with the book's basic premises intact. The book would be much more valuable (to them), they said, if I made it longer, more generic (to attract other specialties), and more expensive. I demurred. Let a gynecologist write a book for gynecologists; my book had a finely focused mission.

Fortunately, someone showed my work to the editors of Oxford University Press, who were happy to issue an inexpensive paperback edition. That slim volume has left its mark. A review of epidemiologic and statistical texts for clinicians, in the *Journal of the Royal Statistical Society*, bemoaned the quality of texts prepared by clinicians, with four exceptions: my slim volume and three more-weighty tomes. A subsequent editorial, in the *Archives of Ophthalmology*, bewailed the dearth of epidemiologic training for ophthalmologists, wistfully recalling "the classic text by Sommer, now long out of print." (I sometimes think of myself in the terms of that editorial: "long out of print!") Thanks to the digital age, that long-out-of-print book has been given a new lease on life. Both the American Academy of Ophthalmology and the International Council of Ophthalmology offer PDF versions of it on their websites.

Discovering the causes of ocular disease and preventing blindness became the core mission guiding my career. Six months before I began my residency at Johns Hopkins, Ed Maumenee had introduced me to a friend of his from Mobile, Alabama, whom he'd known since childhood. Susan Pettis was one of those very special people you meet but rarely. A social worker by training, Susan had been recruited by the American Foundation for Overseas Blind (now Helen Keller International) to direct their newly established blindness prevention program. Susan had recruited Ed to her advisory board, and Ed, in turn, recruited me to be her advisor.

Susan had already decided to focus on childhood blindness in general and vitamin A deficiency in particular. There was growing evidence that vitamin A deficiency, and the blindness it caused, might be much more common than most people had thought. It turned out it was, but we didn't know that then.

Susan's first initiative was to dispatch a faculty member from the University of Illinois to Bangladesh to scout out the problem. Since I'd recently lived in Bangladesh, she asked that I request my colleagues there to assist him. I did. They didn't. Susan expressed exasperation that her consultant couldn't seem to get any cooperation. I got in touch with my connections in Dacca, only to discover that they had decided that Susan's consultant was a competitor, not the person I had asked them to assist. This may have been the least of the misunderstandings we would encounter in a three-decade quest to understand and prevent vitamin A deficiency, and the terrible harm and suffering it caused.

I was convinced that we needed more data about vitamin A and childhood blindness and that only a proper survey of the extent of the problem, and the association of the two conditions, would settle some of our long-standing questions about the matter. I also thought that we could conduct the initial work a bit closer to home. Susan was very supportive, and effective. She obtained funding and permission to conduct a survey in El Salvador and, subsequently, Haiti. She also found a fantastic American expatriate, Peggy McEvoy Doty, who lived in the region and could take care of day-to-day logistics. All I had to do (I was still a full-time Wilmer resident) was fly down a few times, design the surveys and related studies, and analyze and write up the results. My family and I spent one of my winter holiday vacations in El Salvador and another in Haiti.

El Salvador was my first real lesson in the "invisibility" of keratomalacia, a melting of the cornea in children with severe vitamin A deficiency that almost inevitably leads to blindness. It was a lesson I would put to use from then on whenever visiting a country where vitamin A deficiency might be prevalent but underrecognized by the medical profession.

Dr. Esposito, the head ophthalmic honcho in the capital, San Salvador, believed that vitamin A deficiency was a major problem among the poor. He introduced me to the chairman of pediatrics at the main children's hospital.

"No," the head of pediatrics said, "we rarely see children with eye signs of vitamin A deficiency."

I asked, "May I examine the children on the diarrheal and malnutrition wards?"

He did not hesitate in responding, "Of course!"

The third child we encountered was emaciated and lying quietly in bed with his eyes closed. I gently parted his lids: both corneas had melted away. It was classic, severe, blinding vitamin A deficiency. The chief of pediatrics was both chagrined and outraged. He admonished the junior physician for missing the case. The young physician, in turn, yelled at the intern, who in turn yelled at the nurse. I reviewed the chart. The nurse had clearly recorded an abnormality of the child's eyes; none of the physicians had taken notice. We encountered two additional blind children by the time we'd completed our rounds. It was a catalytic moment. With enormous cooperation from all involved, El Salvador carried out the world's first detailed countrywide survey of vitamin A deficiency and xerophthalmia.

Soon after the El Salvador studies concluded, but long before they were published, the World Health Organization and UNICEF convened an international meeting on vitamin A deficiency and xerophthalmia in Jakarta, Indonesia. As one of the few ophthalmologists deeply involved in the problem, I was invited to participate. Indonesian medical officials had long been concerned about the issue, largely because Professor H.A.P.C. Oomen, an internationally renowned Dutch physician, had spent decades in Indonesia (when he wasn't interned in a Japanese prisoner of war camp) documenting the link between vitamin A deficiency and blindness.

I was particularly impressed with the presentation of a young Indonesian biochemist, Muhilal (many Indonesians have only one name), who had recently returned from Liverpool with a doctorate in biochemistry. His carefully conducted study contradicted prevailing wisdom: feeding large amounts of green leafy vegetables to vitamin A–deficient women did not appreciably improve their vitamin A status. Everyone ignored his presentation. In my notes, beside his presentation, I wrote, "Best of Show" (twenty argumentative years later he would prove to be right).

At the meeting, I became increasingly interested in Indonesia. Jill and I longed to continue our overseas adventures. The link between vitamin A deficiency and xerophthalmia was becoming pretty obvious, but important questions remained: How prevalent was the deficiency, and among whom? Why did some children become deficient while others didn't? What was the natural history and clinical course of xerophthalmia? How might it most effectively and practically be prevented and treated? An American colleague also at the conference had spent several years in Indonesia as a medical missionary. I told him of my potential interest in working in the country. He informed me that I was too un-Indonesian: Indonesians, at least those from Central Java (the heart of the country and source of much of its culture and leadership), showed little if any emotion; they remained calm and poker-faced under the most dire conditions. I, on the other hand, constantly emoted and waved my hands about. "For a start," he advised, "keep your hands in your pockets." I tried that for a couple days, but they wouldn't stay there. I decided that I couldn't spend three years with my hands in my pockets.

On the fourth day of the meeting the Indonesian contingent took me aside and "congratulated" me on "winning the sociogram." "What does that mean?" I asked. The response was, "You spoke more often than anyone else." It turned out that the Indonesians were enjoying the antics of this strange but well-meaning American. The next day they asked Susan

Pettis if there was any chance she could persuade me to join them in their vitamin A research. Susan knew of my interest, and soon the deed was done. Jill, Charles, Marni, and I spent the next summer, between my second and third years of residency, in Bandung. I designed three years' worth of studies, to learn all the things (I mistakenly thought) we'd ever need to know about vitamin A deficiency and xerophthalmia.

Pak Tarwotjo, director of the Nutrition Academy in Jakarta, and Professor Sugana, chief of the Cicendo Eye Hospital in Bandung, were my local counterparts. Both were to become close family friends. From the start, Tarwotjo proved his ability to navigate the bureaucracy. To prepare potential designs for our field studies, I needed to make preliminary visits to rural villages, but a foreigner could not visit rural villages without first obtaining permission from the central government (an office locally known as "Sec-Cab"). We handed in my passport and waited for permission. Hearing nothing after two weeks, we simply visited potential field sites. The week I was to return to the U.S. (six weeks after first handing in my passport) Tarwotjo visited Sec-Cab and said to them, "We have canceled plans to visit the field, so Dr. Sommer will not need permission." He emerged with my still unapproved passport.

A year later, with funding from USAID, the Sommer family spent two months in Holland studying Bhasa, the official Indonesian language, and then headed back to Bandung, capital of the mountainous region of West Java, to set up home and office. Jon and Candy Rohde, who had lived next door to us during the tumultuous East Pakistan days, now resided in Central Java, where Jon taught community health for the Rockefeller Foundation. Whenever I left the country, Jill checked to be sure Jon was around for any unexpected pediatric emergencies.

Every overseas experience is different from every other.

Like Bangladesh, Indonesia is overwhelmingly Muslim, but the resemblance pretty much stops there. Bangladesh is flat as a pancake; Indonesia is filled with rolling mountains and active volcanoes. The weekly drive from Bandung to Jakarta was along a narrow, mountain-hugging road that took us over the always fog-enshrouded Puncak Pass before plunging down to the sea-level plains of central Java. Those drives were a study in survival, because exhaust-belching diesel buses would race each other, two abreast, around the curves. Since there was no place for my car to go, other than over a gorge or into the mountainside, I would close my eyes and hope for the best. We were fortunate, but a lot of buses ended up in the gorge.

For all its size and colonial splendor, our house in Bangladesh had been located in a suburban neighborhood and was surrounded by similar compounds. In contrast, our home in Bandung was a more or less conventional single-level ranch-style abode, but it was set back from the road and bordered by an endless field of rice. The only other house we could see was that of our landlord, a wealthy and kindly gold jeweler of Chinese ancestry. "Tuan" ("Uncle," an honorific used in addressing one's seniors) Sunar often walked across the paddy field on weekends to see what "crummy old stuff" ("antiques" in our parlance) we had purchased the week before; artifacts that he and his friends were throwing away (the local rage was to replace traditional furnishings with modern equivalents they'd seen in American television sit-coms).

As always, life overseas was an adventure. Jill and I were sitting in the courtyard one day, when the phone rang. Charles, 8 at the time, picked it up and was addressing the caller. Suddenly we heard him quietly and respectfully say, "Please excuse me, I have to go now, there is a snake in the room." A snake indeed! This one, highly poisonous, had somehow slid in from the paddy field. Our gardener, Anda, approached with great caution, pinned the snake with a broom, and cut its head off with his scythe. From then on we maintained a high level of "snake alert."

Before we had left Indonesia at the end of the planning summer, a senior management team, composed of Tarwotjo, Sugana, and others, had been established. We had also compiled a list of needed equipment and supplies and had detailed the qualifications of the staff that the project would initially employ. When I returned the following year, I proceeded to review the state of preparations. There were none! At least none that were of any value. Sugana had slipped a disc and would remain hospitalized for at least two months. A senior administrator to Tarwotjo had been in a motorcycle accident and had not yet been released from the hospital. The junior administrator had not bothered to order any of the office furniture or supplies but had hired dozens of staff, all of whom appeared to be his relatives.

We started over from scratch—after firing all those who had been recently hired (at my suggestion, the dismissals were blamed on "the American"). Tarwotjo heroically spent three to four days a week in Bandung, returning to Jakarta to run the Nutrition Academy and spend weekends with his family. Proud of what little Bhasa I'd mastered, I insisted that all of our discussions be in their language. Bhasa is among the simplest of languages, with neither tense nor gender. If you want to pluralize a word, you simply say it twice ("anak" for child, "anak anak" for children). After two weeks, Tarwotjo took me aside and asked, "Do you want to improve your Bhasa or get the project done?" I had been hopeless in Bengali but had rationalized that it was not an easy language to master. It seemed I had proved equally hopeless in the far more accessible Bhasa. From then on we carried out most of our business in English.

That is not to say that we always understood one another,

or even that Indonesians always understood their fellow Indonesians, even when they spoke the same language (of the hundreds spoken in Indonesia). One day our senior administrator, Tito, reported that Professor Julie Sulianti, director general of Indonesia's Institute for Health Research and Development—in effect, our boss—had just called and asked that we meet with her at her home in Jakarta at 9:00 the next morning (Saturday). We had no idea why she wanted to meet so urgently, let alone early on a weekend and at her home. We dutifully hit the road at 4:00 a.m. for the long drive to Jakarta (mostly in the dark). We pulled up to her house at 9:00 a.m. sharp and rang the bell. She opened the door (in her house gown), looked at us in bewilderment, and asked, "Was I expecting you?" To this day we have no idea what that call from her office had been about, but it certainly was not a request to meet her early Saturday morning at her home. With usual Indonesian courtesy, she invited us in for breakfast.

Carl Fritz, the only other American on the project—whom I'd hired to help manage logistics and financial affairs—in his 1980 book *Combating Nutritional Blindness in Children*, published a detailed description of our sometimes absurd but always informative miscommunications. These arose, for the most part, from our different cultural backgrounds. He found the weekly management meetings, at which we reviewed progress and finalized plans for the coming week, a rich source of examples and amusement. At one such meeting (devoted to the progress of three field teams surveying the vitamin A status of populations all across Indonesia), I suggested that Team C be in position to survey a particular region on Sumatra the following Monday. "No," my Indonesian colleagues rejoined, "they can't do that on Monday." "Why not?" "They don't sell petrol on Monday." "Of course they sell petrol on Monday." "That's true, but if they have a flat tire they won't be able to have it changed." "Why not?" Silence. It was clear that there was a reason the team couldn't conduct the survey on Monday, but it was a reason that could not be readily explained to an American. It took three such instances before I finally grasped this essential insight, and I never again questioned their hesitations. If it couldn't be done Monday, it would be done Tuesday.

I was, at this time, burning a lot of my personal reserves. In addition to initiating the many investigations, studying for the ophthalmology board examinations I had to take back in the States, teaching the ophthalmology residents in Bandung, and operating on the occasional VIP, I visited Sugana in his hospital room each evening. On one such visit, the third week after settling in, Sugana apologized for what he was about to ask. He was the only retina surgeon in the entire Province of West Java (population 17 million), he explained, and there were twenty-one patients with retinal detachments waiting in the hospital. If I didn't agree to operate on them, they would have to be sent back to their villages. Me? While I'd been well trained at Wilmer to identify retinal detachments and to assist experienced retinal surgeons during an operation, I'd never actually performed the procedure. Besides, the technique I'd learned, freezing the area behind the tear while directly observing the correct location through an indirect ophthalmoscope, was not the technique they used in Bandung. Not to worry, he claimed, they had just obtained a "cryo" (freezing) machine. I agreed, with grave misgivings, because saying no meant certain blindness for these patients.

We scheduled the first five cases for that Saturday. The entire staff turned out to watch. The first patient, a twenty-one-year-old man, was anesthetized with an old style ether cone drip (something I'd never seen before). They plugged in my indirect ophthalmoscope, turned off the lights, and I quickly found and isolated the area of the retinal tear. Now all I needed to do was freeze the outside of the eye immediately behind it. "Cryo," I commanded. It was handed to me. Suddenly everything I was viewing went black!

I cried out, "My indirect has gone off." (Without being able to view the break, I couldn't localize the freeze correctly.)

I was asked, "Which do you want plugged-in, the cryo or the indirect?"

"I need them both."

The response was, "You can't have them both."

I couldn't believe it. "Don't tell me there is only one plug in this entire operating room?"

The silence told me that the answer was yes, there was only one plug.

I stopped the surgery, they turned on the lights, and the anesthesiologist patiently dripped ether as we waited, hopeful that the assistant I'd sent running to the market would return with a multi-plug adapter. One was found, and we finished the five cases without mishap. In the course of the month, all twenty-one patients awaiting surgery received their operation. To my amazement, when we reexamined the patients a year later, all but one had attached retinas and were seeing well. Wilmer colleagues who had gone into retina fellowships had not done more than ten such surgeries during their entire two years of training; they couldn't believe my "good luck" at having gotten to do more than twenty within a month!

Our ambitious series of interlocking studies was, according to a National Academy of Sciences panel who were asked by USAID to review my proposal, grossly *over*ambitious. So much so, that they recommended it not be funded. Had Martin Foreman, then director of USAID's Office of Nutrition, listened to these experts, most of what we now know about the important role vitamin A deficiency plays in causing blindness and death around the world, and how to prevent and treat it, might never have been discovered.

The project consisted of three major investigations related to xerophthalmia:

- Comprehensive examinations of every hospital patient with xerophthalmia (almost exclusively young children), documenting its clinical course, complications, and optimal therapy.
- Repetitive, intensive examination of 4,000 children in 6 rural villages over 18 months. Each exam included a comprehensive physical examination and dietary history to determine the frequency with which xerophthalmia occurred; the goal was to determine why some children became vitamin A deficient while others did not.
- A countrywide survey of 34,000 children and their households across Indonesia, to determine the extent, severity, and location of the problem and what might be its cause in the different parts of the country.

Xerophthalmic corneal ulceration and melting (keratomalacia) is a medical emergency. The 1974 Jakarta meeting had developed treatment recommendations for both the World Health Organization and the International Vitamin A Consultative Group (IVACG). There was substantial evidence from animal studies that the traditional treatment, injection of oily vitamin A, was wholly ineffective; the oily solution sat like a lump under the skin. On the other hand, an injection of vitamin A that was dispersed in water readily entered the circulation and was taken up, and then stored in the liver. Hence, the official recommendation: patients with corneal ulcers and keratomalacia should be treated immediately with an injection of 100,000 IU of water-miscible vitamin A.

After examining our first case of corneal ulceration at the Cicendo Eye Hospital in Bandung, I asked for an ampoule of water-miscible vitamin A for injection. Everyone stared at me. "Water-miscible vitamin A?" Although the official WHO recommendation had been made two years before, there was no water-miscible vitamin A to be had, commercially or otherwise—not just in Indonesia, but anywhere in the world!

The hospital was well stocked with traditional ampoules of oil-miscible vitamin A. Knowing that its injection was unlikely to help, but that a significant amount of vitamin A given by mouth, even in oil, should be absorbed, I took the ampoule, pulled its contents into a syringe, and squirted the vitamin A into the child's mouth. That very afternoon I contacted colleagues at Roche Laboratories and asked them to prepare water-miscible vitamin A injections for clinical use.

To my delight, the child I'd treated with oral, oily vitamin A responded within a few days, and his cornea soon healed. I had the same success with every child I treated that way over the next three months. In the meantime, Roche was formulating, testing, and obtaining the necessary clearances to send water-miscible, injectable vitamin A to Indonesia. By the time Roche's preparation arrived, I was less convinced it was necessary. The oil-miscible form given by mouth seemed to work just fine.

Perhaps I had found a simpler, more practical solution, but I knew we needed data before we would truly know whether oral, oily vitamin A was as effective as an injection of the water-miscible formulation. We launched the first (and what would prove to be the only) randomized trial to compare the effectiveness of these two different approaches for treating severe vitamin A deficiency and its blinding sequelae. I believed that the study could "do no harm," because I'd seen how well oral dosing had worked when there was no rational alternative.

Every child we encountered who had corneal ulcers from vitamin A deficiency was randomized, by lottery, to receive one of the two treatments (oily vitamin A by mouth or watery vitamin A by injection) on day one, while both groups received a second oral dose on the second day (to "top up" their vitamin A reserves). The primary outcome of interest was the clinical response, that is, the proportion in which the ulcers began to improve and the time it took for their corneal ulcers to heal. The clinical response was identical in the two groups: no child got worse, and the ulcers healed with equal rapidity. Muhilal, with his freshly minted doctorate in the biochemistry of vitamin A, documented that both treatments had the same, critical, biochemical response, supporting the equivalency of the clinical responses. He employed a new technique, which he had developed while he was in Liverpool, that was far more reflective of vitamin A status than the older techniques that were then still widely in use. This was as good as clinical research ever gets!

Our simple, unanticipated trial had enormous practical implications. Oily vitamin A was cheap and widely available and could be safely administered orally by anyone. A thoughtful person (a teacher, health aide, village head-man) without any medical training could safely treat a child who might otherwise soon become permanently blind. Water-miscible, injectable vitamin A, while effective, was less stable and far more expensive, required a sterile needle and syringe to administer, and could only be given by trained medical personnel. It also was not readily available anywhere in the world.

The chapter should have ended with this happy finding and its implementation. The policy implications of this simple clinical trial seemed pretty straightforward. The trial was published in the peer-reviewed literature and presented at the next IVACG meeting. I formally recommended that we change the WHO/IVACG recommendation to the oral administration of oil-miscible vitamin A for the treatment of xerophthalmia or any other evidence of serious vitamin A deficiency.

Not for the first (or the last) time, however, I discovered that once members of an "expert body" have spoken, they tend to be wedded to their opinion. The "vitamin A nutrition community" was entirely unmoved by our study.

I countered with statements along the line of "But data are data!"

Someone challenged, "A child could spit out the oily vitamin A."

"No, they can't spit it out; it is oily and sticks to their mouth. Besides, it worked in every child we studied."

Someone else objected, "Parents like to see their children receive an injection."

There was some truth in this statement, as people had come to see injections as cures. But, since the only vitamin A preparations readily available were oily, and their injection did absolutely no good, we would be recommending a useless treatment instead of a simpler and far more effective one, and a lot of children would suffer the consequences.

This "expert panel" reached a crazy compromise. The original recommendation of water-miscible vitamin A by injection (still rarely available) was retained, but a footnote in tiny print was added saying that oily vitamin A could be used by mouth if the water-miscible injectable preparation was unavailable. I knew that few health personnel anywhere in the world read footnotes or fine print, and that there was no water-miscible vitamin A in the countries that most needed it. This "revision" was worthless. It simply solidified the importance of an injection, and if all that was available was oily vitamin A (almost inevitably the case), then that's what would be (uselessly) injected.

Blatant, obtuse obstruction can be frustrating; worse, it has led more than one investigator to lose interest in translating a finding into practice. Alternatively, you can grit your teeth and keep plugging. I plugged on, but it took five years of advocacy before oral dosing with vitamin A was recommended as an acceptable "alternative" to injectable water-miscible vitamin A, and another five years of effort before injectable vitamin A became the footnote. After a long decade, data finally guided policy and practice.

IF YOU THINK YOU'RE RIGHT, KEEP PUSHING

Never doubt that a single individual can change the
world. Indeed, it is the only thing that ever has.

MARGARET MEAD

I left Indonesia in 1979 with plans to launch a randomized trial to determine whether large doses of oral vitamin A given just twice a year could prevent blinding xerophthalmia among young children. If it could, the impact
could be enormous. It would make a global blindness-prevention program financially and practically feasible.

Our surveys had revealed that xerophthalmia was extremely common in Aceh Province, on the island of Sumatra. It would therefore be the perfect place for the study. It
took two years to assemble the funds and another year to
obtain government clearance and to build the teams and in-
frastructure needed to carry it out.

The Indonesian government was by then committed to
a vitamin A supplementation program. Purposely denying
children vitamin A, by randomly assigning them to receive
a placebo, which could lead to blindness, was completely off
the table. However, the government's planned intervention
program was to be rolled out over five years, covering an ad-

ditional one-fifth of all villages in each succeeding year. So, we asked that the government allow us to randomize the order in which the villages were added to the program. That way, we could conduct a properly randomized trial, comparing villages randomly assigned to be in the program with neighboring villages randomly assigned to join the program subsequently, without interfering with the coverage the government hoped to achieve.

Our approach abandoned the traditional use of placebos in the control villages. Placebos are most critical when a study's outcome of interest is subjective, like a patient's perceived level of pain, wellness, or improvement. Such subjective outcomes can be influenced by the patient's and the researcher's expectations regarding the treatment. Blindness, or lack thereof, is a "hard" clinical manifestation, about as hard as it gets, short of death. The placebo-less approach was also the only design for which the Indonesian government would provide its ethical approval. While I did not see the absence of a traditional placebo as a significant shortcoming of the study, later opponents did!

Just before launching the project, I had a sudden, unexpected (and dramatic) cause to alter its primary objective. Every member of our group refers to this observation, one that changed our lives and careers, and more importantly, global health policy, as the "holy cow moment." (In honesty, "cow" was not the noun I originally uttered.)

Late one afternoon in 1982, over the Christmas holidays, when patients rarely came in for cataract or glaucoma surgery, I was poring over computer printouts of the (by then "old") Indonesian study in which we'd examined village children every three months for eighteen months. The purpose of that study had been to determine whether certain attributes (diet, illnesses) distinguished those children who later developed xerophthalmia from those who didn't.

In flipping through the printouts, I noticed something entirely unexpected. Children found to have night blindness or Bitot's spots (early symptoms and signs of xerophthalmia) on one examination were less likely than non-xerophthalmic children to present for their follow-up examination three months later. It turned out that children with signs of "mild xerophthalmia" were more likely than non-xerophthalmic children to have died in the interim. I rang up my statistician, Joanne Katz (now a senior professor at Johns Hopkins), that evening and asked her to come in over the weekend to formally rerun the data, this time focusing on mortality as the outcome of interest.

The formal, computerized analysis confirmed my back-of-the-envelope calculations: children with night blindness had died at three times the rate of children with normal eyes; children with Bitot's spots (slightly more vitamin A deficient) died at six times the rate; and children with both night blindness and Bitot's spots (more deficient still) died at nearly nine times the rate of their unaffected peers. We were stunned by the apparent strength of the association between vitamin A deficiency and childhood mortality!

In science, certainty is hard to demonstrate. While we knew that vitamin A deficiency *might* have been responsible for this excess childhood mortality, we also realized that the association might *not* have been causal; vitamin A status could have been "tracking" other characteristics, which might explain this apparent association. Those who were vitamin A deficient might also have been more malnourished, or younger, or suffering from other conditions we hadn't identified that accounted for their increased mortality. So we stratified the children by those characteristics ("confounders"). But, even when we compared only children of the same age who had normal protein-energy nutrition and no history of respiratory illness or diarrhea at the time of the prior examination, the results remained consistently unchanged. Every group displayed the same pattern: the more severe the vitamin A deficiency, the greater the mortality.

These surprising results, when published in a lead article in the *Lancet*, were greeted with less than a yawn. No one bothered to write a single letter to the editor either for or against the findings and their implications; no one rushed off to conduct a study to prove or disprove them. The results and implications were so at odds with conventional wisdom about the causes of childhood deaths in the developing world that they were entirely ignored. The vast majority of deaths were "known" to be caused by infectious diseases, exacerbated by protein-energy malnutrition and the miserable, unhygienic conditions in which these children lived.

Our team, however, was energized by these findings, and we took the opposite tack. These were results that demanded further exploration. The planned blindness-prevention trial in Aceh was redirected to have mortality reduction as its primary outcome. Children in the 250 villages randomized to receive the large-dose vitamin A twice a year died at only two-thirds the rate of the children in the 250 control villages. This report, also published as the lead article in the *Lancet* (and accompanied by a supportive editorial), received a far different response than the preceding, observational study had; instead of being ignored, it met with an outpouring of hostile and disbelieving letters to the editor. Orthodoxy had been challenged a second time, by an unconventionally large, randomized clinical trial.

The depth and breadth of the hostility caught me entirely by surprise. Prior experience (mine and others) should have prepared me for the response. Over a century ago, Virchow noted that "experts" tend to respond to new paradigms in the same way people grieve: the initial response is denial. Subsequent stages progress through hostility to, finally, grudging acceptance. Why new (if startling) results that might help humanity should be greeted as bad news was another matter. You can eventually force the expert community to change their thinking, but only if you undertake more studies, stimulate others to do the same, and finally bury conventional wisdom with data.

You also need to monitor the publications of others to insure that they are generating and interpreting their own data appropriately! One well-executed study published in the *New England Journal of Medicine* reported essentially the same overall results we (repeatedly) had. But, unlike many of our studies, in which we'd consistently found a 50 percent reduction in deaths from measles among those given vitamin A, they reported no such relationship. An accompanying editorial emphasized this apparent discrepancy. Yet, the data provided in their publication listed 12 deaths in the placebo group and 7 deaths in the vitamin A group, about as close to a 50 percent reduction in mortality as one could reasonably expect in a community-based randomized trial. What they had mistaken for the absence of impact was the absence of a statistically significant difference, which was not present, because the sample size was too small to guarantee that the relatively large clinical difference they observed wasn't a chance event. What they (and the editorial writer) should have concluded was that they had found *exactly* the same impact on measles that we had but, because of their small sample size, the difference wasn't statistically significant.

By 1992 there were sufficiently supportive trials from so many countries that I hoped this vexing debate could finally be brought to an end. I invited two dozen experts in nutrition, early childhood mortality, and other disciplines to spend a week reviewing and assessing all the relevant, available data. At the end of the five days, it was unanimously agreed that what had traditionally been considered "mild" or "early" vitamin A deficiency (levels of deficiency associated with night blindness and Bitot's spots) was in fact "severe," already compromising a child's ability to survive an infectious episode. The assembled experts agreed to return home and report the results of our deliberations in their local medical journals.

Control of vitamin A deficiency is now a global policy of both the World Health Organization and UNICEF, and there are now vitamin A deficiency control programs in nearly seventy countries around the world. The World Bank and the economists of the Copenhagen Consensus rank vitamin A supplementation as one of the most cost-effective of all health interventions, with the potential for saving the sight and the lives of a million children every year.

This rather astounding global impact began when my wife and I decided to spend a few more years in the developing world. It was propelled by a compulsively conducted investigation carried out for other reasons entirely and was vaulted to a new level by a chance observation (one holiday evening) of an unexpected outcome lurking among the data. But in the end it depended upon dogged determination to prove that data are important and that clinically compelling data should give rise to appropriate global policy.

TAKE THE LONG VIEW

The major factors that brought health to mankind were epidemiology, sanitation, vaccination, refrigeration, and screened windows.

RICHARD D. LAMM

Like most people who keep their nose to the grindstone, I had achieved a modest amount of attention within my limited circles. But I was also viewed as an epidemiological and ophthalmological iconoclast. Getting tagged as an iconoclast can be a double-edged sword; it allows people to dismiss your perspectives, but it also attracts people who feel that a different perspective might be exactly what's needed. How else to explain my being tapped, in 1990, to be dean of the Johns Hopkins (now Bloomberg) School of Public Health? Definitely an unusual job for an ophthalmologist. One Johns Hopkins University trustee (who did not know me) was heard to moan to another, "An ophthalmologist as dean of public health? Couldn't they find anyone better?"

Shortly after ascending to this administrative position, I unintentionally rattled my new colleagues, fellow deans on the board of the Association of Schools of Public Health (ASPH). Their twice-a-year meetings were extremely formal affairs, with the deans of the then twenty-two accredited schools of public health (at the time, only American schools) sitting around a large table listening to rather boring, long-winded committee reports. Their associate deans sat behind them, and their flag bearers, still farther behind. A mini-UN in appearance and tone, this assembly accomplished nothing of importance, as far as I could tell. I also sensed considerable tension between a number of the deans, who seemed to consider one another as competitors, or worse. To me, the greater purpose of public health was taking a back seat to formality, personalities, estrangement, and turf. Also, these meetings weren't much fun!

Not only did these ritualistic meetings serve little discernible purpose, but they were held in the most depressing venues—often seedy downtown hotels. I have long believed that, to a reasonable point, people feel only as good as their surroundings; if these meetings were to become more effective, we needed to change both their organization and their venue.

I suggested we try something different. How about a three-day, informal retreat in a nice setting, off-season and some place not too costly (we were, after all, public health people, not Park Avenue clinicians). Let's bring our spouses and partners and get to know one another, as fellow deans swimming in the same pool and beset by the same problems. Someone, to my surprise, exclaimed, "That's a brilliant idea." I remember remarking to a colleague nearby, "If an informal retreat in a pleasant setting is a 'brilliant idea,' public health is in even worse shape than I had thought."

The first retreat, held off-season at Rosario in the San Juan Islands, proved immensely productive and enjoyable. The deans came to better know one another; they shared frustrations and helpful suggestions and planned a pallet of future initiatives. This now-annual event has deans enthusiastically tackling the needs of public health and seeing their schools as part of a larger purpose.

I also noted that ASPH had been in the habit of adopting every worthy cause that came its way, from increasing NIH funding to more equitable access to health care for the poor. The intent was noble, but the "embrace everything worthy" approach was not helping anyone. ASPH is a small organization with a tiny budget. I thought we would do better to focus on those issues most critical to making our schools more effective and should choose those causes unlikely to be championed by larger and more powerful institutions. Supporting increased NIH funding was important, but we could add little to the powerful and diverse constituency already beating that drum.

I suggested that we hire a professional lobbyist, to better guide our efforts. The immediate response was that "public health doesn't get in bed with lobbyists!" So I decided that the Johns Hopkins School of Public Health would hire a lobbyist. Robert C. Embry, the insightful president of the Baltimore-based Abell Foundation, agreed to pay the costs of the lobbyist when I assured him that the efforts would strengthen the school and public health in Baltimore. The outcome was remarkably successful. People soon noticed that influencing legislation could truly make a university more effective. In time, the deans on the ASPH board changed their minds, so the Hopkins public health lobbyists expanded their scope to serve the whole association.

Years later, I became ASPH's president, at a time when it had become apparent that the organization needed to be entirely restructured. We hired a full-time, well-known public health luminary, Harrison Spencer, to lead the organization and serve as its chief spokesman. These changes were not easily made, but their impact has been transformational.

Public health has long received far too little public attention and support (its public heyday was nearly a century ago). In part, this is because the public health community is largely composed of deeply compassionate professionals sympathetic to underdogs and lost causes; they are not perceived as essential to the well-being of the average citizen. During a luncheon address to the leadership of the U.S. Public Health Service Commissioned Corps, of which I'd been a member when at the CDC, I asked (rhetorically, and with some trepidation), "Why are we content to be seen as poor doctors for poor people?" and, "Why isn't the Surgeon General [head of the corps] seen as the physician for all Americans?"

When composing my remarks, I had worried that they might cause offense; instead, they received a standing ovation! I was stunned. Senior public health officers in the room urged me to publish the talk. It appeared in *Public Health Reports*, titled "W(h)ither Public Health?" Clearly, many public health practitioners were ready for changes in the way we went about our mission and interacted with the public.

Public health is about the collective and intertwined health of us all. Effective global health leadership is distinguished by logical, flexible approaches to solving critically important health problems; by framing meaningful questions and designing creative ways to provide their answers; by seeking worthy causes, but only those that can be practically addressed and whose solution will make a palpable difference; and by approaches, conclusions, and applications that are based on data, driven by passion, and implemented through persistence.

Straightforward epidemiologic investigation and reasoning remain the core of important health-related discovery and the design of effective global health policies and programs whose goal, as in the motto of the Bloomberg School, is "protecting health and saving lives, millions at a time."

In this book, I have looked at global (public) health through the lens of my own experiences, not because they are particularly noteworthy but because they are the ones I know best. I hope this personal tale has successfully illustrated something of the potential breadth and depth of cultural adventures, intellectual challenges, discoveries, and contributions to human welfare offered by a career in epidemiology and a life in global health.

There is still much ill in the world. Some of that ill will be lessened by those of you who choose public health as a career. Can you make a difference? Unquestionably, *if* you are guided by what most interests and excites you, seize opportunity at every turn, see data as the critical foundation of decisionmaking, persevere when you know your data are honest and reliable, lead an ethical life, and unceasingly strive to change clinical practice and health policy for the better.

EPILOGUE

Life is either a daring adventure, or nothing.

HELEN KELLER

|||||||||||||||||||||||||||||||||||||||||||||||||||||||||||||||||||||||||||||||||||||||||||||||||||||||||||||||||||||||||||||||||||

I spend a good deal of my time these days informally mentoring those who drop by my office for advice. They may be entering students or a young professor or even a chair or dean. Their main question is nearly always the same: "What should I do with my life?" My answer is always the same: "What would you *like* to do with your life?" After their first quizzical look, I respond with my four favorite aphorisms (a few of which you've already been exposed to in this treatise).

The first and perhaps most important, is attributed to Yogi Berra: "If there's a fork in the road, take it." I have no idea what *he* meant by that, but I have given it my own interpretation. Life is filled with "forks in the road," opportunities that call for a choice in direction. All too often, smart, goal-oriented individuals find their ability to make these choices frozen by the number of their options and the importance they attribute to them. You can't do randomized trials on forks in the road. You have to choose between them. My best advice is to choose the fork that excites you the most, the one that is most likely to keep you up at night thinking. That's the path you will most likely find productive and fulfilling. And if that turns out not to be the case, don't worry—life is filled with forks in the road, and another fork will soon come along.

The second, and related, insight to live by was offered by Woody Allen: "Eighty percent of success is showing up." If you don't show up and aren't engaged, you won't encounter those forks in the road, nor will you be thinking deeply and innovatively (most often when sleeping or walking up a mountain path) in ways that lead to insights, insights that sometimes change you and change the world.

Hence the third important aphorism: Louis Pasteur's "Chance favors the prepared mind." The most-cited example of this phenomenon, perhaps, is Fleming's discovery of penicillin. Microbiologists (including Fleming, it must be mentioned) had been frustrated for years by the fact that bacteria would not grow on culture plates adjacent to fungal contaminants. They would hurl the plates away in frustration. Until the day that Fleming finally asked the (now obvious) question: Why don't bacteria grow when adjacent to penicillium mold? Answer: Because the mold secreted a product that killed the bacteria—the first antibiotic was discovered. While I am not in Fleming's league, my pursuing distant, ghostly forms to a cemetery at four in the morning, and recognizing my discovery's practical implications, or my pondering why some Indonesian children were less likely than others to show up for their next examination, meant I was open to opportunities for discovery that unexpected events provided. If an experiment turns out exactly as expected, you haven't truly learned anything. It's the right angle, unexpected results that provide new insights and directions, even if they put you at odds with established wisdom and those who hold to it.

And that leads us to the last aphorism: "Persistence pays." Had we not repeated, and helped others to repeat, our vitamin A supplementation trials, we'd never have established the basis for what is widely regarded today as a core child survival strategy. When younger colleagues grew angry at the negative responses to another one of our well-conducted trials, I would reassure them that we would one day prevail, by "burying the naysayers with data."

Get engaged, choose the most personally interesting of your options, think deeply and innovatively, and bury them with data.